With Compassion Toward Some

Homosexuality and Social Work in America

With Compassion Toward Some

Homosexuality and Social Work in America

Edited by

Robert Schoenberg and Richard S. Goldberg
with David A. Shore

With Compassion Toward Some: Homosexuality and Social Work in America was originally published in 1984 by The Haworth Press, Inc. It has also been published as *Journal of Social Work and Human Sexuality*, Volume 2, Numbers 2/3, Winter 1983/Spring 1984.

Harrington Park Press
New York • London

ISBN 0-918393-14-0

Published by

Harrington Park Press, Inc.
28 East 22 Street
New York, New York 10010-6194

EUROSPAN/Harrington
3 Henrietta Street
London WC2E 8LU England

Harrington Park Press, Inc., is a subsidiary of The Haworth Press, Inc., 28 East 22 Street, New York, New York 10010-6194.

With Compassion Toward Some: Homosexuality and Social Work in America was originally published in 1984 by The Haworth Press, Inc., under the title *Homosexuality and Social Work*. It has also been published as *Journal of Social Work and Human Sexuality*, Volume 2, Numbers 2/3, Winter 1983/Spring 1984.

Library of Congress Cataloging in Publication Data

Main entry under title:

With compassion toward some.

    Rev. ed. of: Homosexuality and social work. c1984.
    "Also been published as Journal of social work and human sexuality, volume 2, numbers 2/3, Winter 1983/Spring 1984"—T.p. verso.
    Includes bibliographies.
    1. Social work with homosexuals—United States—Addresses, essays, lectures.
I. Schoenberg, Robert. II. Goldberg, Richard S. III. Shore, David A. IV. Homosexuality and social work.
HV1449.W58   1985   361.8   85-5838
ISBN 0-918393-14-0 (pbk.)

CONTENTS

II. LIFE PROBLEMS

III. PROFESSIONAL ISSUES

ABOUT THE EDITORS

Robert Schoenberg, ACSW, is Program Advisor in the Office of Student Life and Counselor in the University Counseling Service at the University of Pennsylvania in Philadelphia. Both positions involve working with and on behalf of lesbian and gay students. Mr. Schoenberg has also been serving as lecturer at the University of Pennsylvania School of Social Work and has taught in the University's undergraduate leadership training program. He has written several articles and made presentations at many professional meetings. Prior to his return to academic life, he worked for several years as social worker and social work supervisor in the area of mental retardation and as a consultant for several special mental health/mental retardation projects. Mr. Schoenberg has volunteered considerable time with a variety of organizations, including serving for seven years on the Board of Directors of the Eromin Center in Philadelphia (three years as Board Chairperson). He is currently serving as a member of the Steering Committee of the Philadelphia AIDS Task Force.

Richard S. Goldberg, MSS, is on the staff of the Institute for Human Identity, New York City. He is former head of the Gay Program at Episcopal Community Services in Philadelphia. He is a graduate of the School of Social Work and Social Research of Bryn Mawr College. In addition to practicing social work, he has contributed many articles to the popular gay press, including *The Advocate*, the *Philadelphia Gay News*, the *New York Native*, and *Christopher Street*.

David A. Shore, MPA, ACSW, is the Associate Director, Accreditation Program for Psychiatric Facilities, Joint Commission on Accreditation of Hospitals and Founding Editor, *Journal of Social Work & Human Sexuality*.

CONTRIBUTORS

Ted R. Bohn, MSW
Rutgers Law School
Newark, NJ

Beverly Decker, MSW
Psychotherapist and Supervisor
Institute for Human Identity
Psychotherapist in Private Practice
New York, NY

Teresa DeCrescenzo, MSW
Clinical Social Worker in Private
    Practice
Chair, California Board
    of Behavioral Science Examiners
Los Angeles, CA

Jack Louis DeVine, MA
Coordinator of Family Support
    Services
Lesbian and Gay Community Services
Minneapolis, MN

Harvey L. Gochros, DSW
Professor and Chair, MSW Program
University of Hawaii
School of Social Work
Honolulu, HI

Morgan Gwenwald, MSW
Coordinator of Direct Services
Senior Action in a Gay Environment
New York, NY

Joyce Lewis, MSS
Associate Professor
Graduate School of Social Work
    and Social Research
Bryn Mawr College
Bryn Mawr, PA

Alice E. Messing, MA, Ph.D.
    (Cand.)
Health Care Management Consultant
Formerly, Executive Director
Philadelphia Community Health
    Alternatives
Philadelphia, PA

Robert Schoenberg, MSW, ACSW
Lecturer, School of Social Work
Program Advisor and Counselor
    for Gay/Lesbian Students
University of Pennsylvania
Philadelphia, PA

Roger K. Stephens, MSSA, ACSW
Director of Social Work
Graduate Hospital
Philadelphia, PA

Tacie L. Vergara, MSW
Director of Youth Services
Eromin Center, Inc.
Philadelphia, PA

Marta Ann Zehner, MSS
Associate Director
Women Organized Against Rape
Philadelphia, PA

Preface

Homosexuality and Social Work was prepared to assist social workers and social service agencies in helping lesbians and gay men with the problems they face in their lives. It is the third volume in the *Journal of Social Work & Human Sexuality* series of thematic issues geared at focusing on special populations. Like its predecessors, *Social Work & Child Sexual Abuse* and *Human Sexuality in Medical Social Work,* this present volume makes the point that there are issues and concerns that are particularly idiosyncratic to this special population. Also, like its predecessors, this present text powerfully makes the point that the field of social work is well suited to service the homosexually-oriented.

As I review proposals for future thematic issues, it becomes more and more clear that any list of special populations or sexual minorities is arbitrary. There can be no final or ultimate list and any subset of activities or beliefs or preferences can become the basis for the claim for minority status. As John Gagnon has pointed out, "all of these minorities raise serious moral and psychological questions about the limits of the 'normal' and our capacity to understand others, to move ourselves inside someone else and experience the world as that person does." To deny or to ignore the oppressed status of minority group members is to ignore the reality of their external environments. When it comes to issues of human sexuality, the larger society has for too long defined "healthy" sexuality. This situation is changing as professionals become more sensitive to the need to develop strategies that can help oppressed minority groups in their struggle with personal and social problems.

It has always been my belief that social workers need to be, and are appropriately well positioned to be on the forefront of the struggle for sexual equality. With *Homosexuality and Social Work* we have gone beyond the bulk of the literature which consists primarily of attempts to show that homosexual individuals are somehow physiologically abnormal or psychologically unhealthy. This anti-homosexualism as it was called, or homophobia as it is called, is well attended to in this volume. Indeed, *Homosexuality and So-*

cial Work provides the necessary conceptual marriage to work effectively with any special population—it addresses the affective, cognitive and skills components of working with and for lesbians and gay men. It is my hope that those who study this work will feel better prepared to provide the same kind of quality care to the homosexually-oriented that they are now providing to their other clients.

David A. Shore

Introduction

This text is about social workers helping lesbians and gay men with problems they face in their lives. In many instances, the problems which gay men and lesbians face are either the direct result of or exacerbated by negative attitudes toward homosexuality and the consequent hostile or discriminatory actions directed toward homosexuals.

It is our view that the field of social work is uniquely suited to serving lesbians and gay men. After all, social work has a dual focus—on people and the social environment in which they live. Social workers are concerned with interactions between individuals and society. Work at this "boundary" involves helping individuals understand and cope with their environment and advocating for societal change aimed at improving peoples' lives. The problems presented by gay men and lesbians can be addressed most effectively using this approach.

Many of the articles in this collection discuss homophobia—the fear of homosexuality—and the resultant mistreatment and oppression of lesbians and gay men. This fear is widespread and deep-seated in our society. Thus few—heterosexual or homosexual—have escaped it. Not only have homosexuals been the targets of homophobic behavior but internalized homophobia has resulted in some gay men and lesbians having diminished self-images and inaccurate views that their problems are idiosyncratic. Social workers who understand these dynamics can help lesbians and gay men recognize homophobia and develop effective strategies for confronting and overcoming the difficulties of being homosexual in a predominantly heterosexual world. At the same time, social workers can work toward changes in society's negative attitudes and oppressive acts.

Gay men and lesbians appear in the full range of agencies and settings in which social workers work. Some are poor, some are handicapped, some are old, some are incarcerated. Naturally, these clients have the needs that their heterosexual counterparts have in the settings where social workers encounter them. But there are also profound differences. Their sexual orientation often has a great effect on the way they view their social environment, its role in creating and sustaining their situation, and its willingness to help them. As we wrote in an earlier article:

> What distinguishes gay social work is not that it is services provided by social workers (homosexual or not) to gay and lesbian clients; it is the adaptations in the provision of services necessitated by society's negative attitudes toward homosexuality and by homosexuals' responses to those attitudes.[1]

This collection expands on that view by identifying specific adaptations appropriate to specific settings and by discussing the theoretical underpinnings of those adaptations.

It would be impossible in a work of this size to explore the full range of settings and situations in which lesbians and gay men find themselves or all of the theoretical bases of social work with homosexuals. We herewith identify but a handful of the many topics which space does not permit us to include, subjects which we hope will be studied in other forums.

—WOMEN AND RACIAL MINORITIES—Gay men of color and lesbians, both white and of color, have special concerns and needs. For one thing, their self-definition as homosexual may be different from that of white gay men. For example, women often report becoming aware of their homosexual feelings later in life than do gay men; for black men, homosexuality is often associated only with the passive sex role. The concept of sexual orientation which is prevalent (and used by us) may be a white male, middle-class definition. Lesbians and gay men of color experience double or even triple discrimination in our society. These individuals may identify primarily with the group most discriminated against. Thus for lesbians or gay men of color, the self-definition as homosexual may be secondary. An understanding of the differences and the particular needs of gay men of color and lesbians and the interventions and services required of social workers is a rich area for further work.

—LESBIANS/GAY MEN AS PARENTS—The fact that lesbians and gay men are parents is often forgotten or denied. Homosexual parents have all the same needs as heterosexual parents; they also have particular concerns. These need to be further considered.

—ETHICAL CONSIDERATIONS—All of the usual social work guidelines and prohibitions apply—especially those pertaining to working with disadvantaged, vulnerable populations. It seems, however, that in certain ethical realms, gay and lesbian clients merit special, if not unique, consideration. Among these realms are self-determination and confidentiality. This needs to be further explored and discussed.

—INDIRECT PRACTICE—The focus of most of the articles in the collection is direct practice. This is appropriate since direct practice is the activity in which most social workers are engaged. But gay and lesbian clients can be served well by interventions at other levels. Though these indirect practice processes are mentioned in some of the articles, more particular and extensive attention is required. Specifically, these practice processes are: administration, policy development, community organization, advocacy/lobbying/politics.

This volume is divided into three sections. Each section offers a particular perspective on social work with gay men and lesbians as individuals and in communities.

The four articles in the first section are concerned with life stages and statuses—families, youth, couples, aging. These are stages and statuses experienced by homosexuals and heterosexuals alike, but, as noted earlier, the sameness is accompanied by significant difference. Social workers need to expand their knowledge of these phenomena as they are experienced by lesbians and gay men. It requires a cross-cultural sort of understanding. Familiarity with the nature and content of their gay clients' experiences will enhance social workers' interventions.

The contributions of Vergara (youth) and Gwenwald (aging) provide dramatic examples of the sameness/difference and double discrimination themes discussed earlier. Homosexual youth and homosexual elderly share disadvantages and ageist discrimination with their heterosexual age-mates, but have particular concerns and needs because of society's view of and reaction to their sexual orientation. These two practice-based articles concentrate on the development and provision of innovative services within the context of gay/lesbian agencies.

The articles by DeVine and Decker offer new applications of established theoretical bases for working with families and couples. Couples and families have always been among the most common units receiving social work services. Little attention has been given to providing services to homosexual couples and to families with homosexual members. The provision of these services can take place within any social agency, including traditional ones.

While the articles in Section I concentrate on life stages, the three articles in Section II focus on life problems—medical, psychological, social—which traverse age and stage. The dangerous and insidious nature of homophobia is particularly evident in these chapters. The problems discussed—inadequate health care (Messing, Schoenberg, and Stephens), alcoholism (Zehner and Lewis), and violence (Bohn)—affect all groups of people. But when they hit gay men and lesbians, it seems, they hit harder. The articles suggest that, all other factors being equal, lesbians and gay men are more prone to being the victims of poor health care, alcoholism, and violence than their heterosexual counterparts.

Though each of the articles in Sections I and II discusses implications and provides recommendations for social work practice, the components of Section III concern themselves specifically with the profession and resources for practitioners. DeCrescenzo brings to light the attitudes of members of the various helping professions toward homosexuals. Her findings about social workers are particularly interesting and useful. Gochros discusses teaching social workers about gay men and lesbians, their particular concerns and needs.

The social work profession has made considerable progress in the last ten years in recognizing and learning how to meet the needs of lesbians and gay men. The National Association of Social Workers has taken official positions favoring equal rights and equal treatment for gay men and lesbians, discrimination on the basis of sexual orientation is prohibited in the *Code of Ethics* and other NASW documents, and a standing committee is working to monitor and improve policies and procedures affecting lesbians and gay men.[2] A Gay and Lesbian Task Force has been working within the Council on Social Work Education, non-discrimination on the basis of sexual orientation is included in revised accreditation standards, and the Curriculum Policy Statement adopted in 1982 includes the following:

> The curriculum must provide content on ethnic minorities of color and women. It should include content on other special population groups relevant to the program's mission or location and, in particular, groups that have been consistently affected by social, economic, and legal bias or oppression. Such groups include, but are not limited to, those distinguished by age, religion, disablement, sexual orientation and culture.[3]

These efforts have been very important but much more needs to be done. Social work practitioners and students need to become familiar with the particular needs and concerns of lesbians and gay men and to learn effective strategies for intervention. We believe this collection of articles can contribute to that process.

Robert Schoenberg
Richard S. Goldberg

NOTES

1. Richard S. Goldberg and Robert Schoenberg, "Defining Gay Social Work: Beginning with Beginnings." *CATALYST* Volume III Number 4 (1981) p. 81.

2. For more information, contact the National Committee on Lesbian and Gay Issues, NASW, 7981 Eastern Avenue, Silver Spring, MD 20910.

3. For more information, contact the Gay and Lesbian Task Force, CSWE, Suite 501, 111 Eighth Avenue, New York, NY 10011.

I

Life Stages and Statuses

A Systemic Inspection
of Affectional Preference Orientation
and the Family of Origin

ABSTRACT. Clinical intervention with families of origin where a child has a same-gender affectional preference orientation has led to the synthesis of a five-staged developmental model reflective of the systemic changes that the family undergoes as it attempts to cope with the affectional preference issue. The first three stages of the process attempt to maintain homeostatic function, whereas, the latter two bring about resolution and integrate the child back into the system. The three system variables that have a profound effect on the outcome of the family's movements are cohesion, regulative structure and family themes. Strategies for positive intervention are presented.

The sequential, systemic, adaptative process and intervention strategies being presented are based on the premise that same-gender affectional preference orientation becomes a major crisis for the family system because: (1) there are no rules in the family system appropriate to handle the behavior, (2) there are no roles in the family specific to the issue into which the family members can fit, (3) there is no constructive language available to describe the issue, (4) there are strong negative family and cultural proscriptions against homosexual behavior, (5) the cohesive element, regulative structure and themes within the family system become critical forces against adaptation.

This model assumes that foreclosure on the process can and does occur at each developmental stage with social and psychological loss to the members of the family system. The model has been

---

The author gratefully acknowledges the extensive contributions of Douglas Elwood and Judith K. Scott in the synthesis of the model.

9

synthesized from intervention with families who were Caucasian, intact, lower upper to middle income with Christian and European ethnic focus. These factors may limit its applicability.

In discussing the family system the term "focal member" is used to refer to the person whose nonheterosexual feelings are emerging or actively being acted upon and thus impacting the family system of origin.

CRITICAL FACTORS AND SYSTEM ADAPTATION

The family's systemic adaptation to affectional preference issues can be viewed as a passage through a sequence of developmental stages. Not all families are willing to undertake the process nor do all families complete the process. Because the family system varies from constellation to constellation families do not move from one developmental stage to the next stage with the same rapidity or internal stresses. Completion of the process, that is reaching the stage of integration, does not signify that the affectional preference orientation will no longer present issues for family resolution but rather that these issues will be resolved in a manner that is respectful, open and supportive to all of the family members. It is to this end that all strategic interventions should be directed.

The critical systemic factors of cohesion, regulative structure and family themes that govern the family's movements in the resolution of affectional preference issues are those same factors that promote or hinder movement in any adaptive process.

Cohesion is the distance or closeness of the emotional bonding that occurs between family members and the degree of autonomy that this bond affords members within the system. The cohesive element spans a continuum from extremely high cohesion, "enmeshed," where members are so closely bonded that little autonomy exists, to "disengaged" where the members experience very little affectional bonding and family solidarity.

The regulative structure is composed of the spoken rules, the unspoken rules and the role expectations that serve as a mechanism for the control of the members within the system. It spans a continuum from "rigid" where rules and roles are not viewed as readily changeable to "chaotic" where rules and roles are ill-defined or unpredictable.

Family themes have as their focus the projection of the family system to outside environments from which the family can assume a position with respect to its on-going interactions with these environments. These positions thus in turn directly affect internal movements within the system as they define family strategy and answer two important questions: "Who are we as a family?" and "What ought we as a family do about it?" Much of the family's ability to move toward an integrative position in reference to the gay or lesbian member will be reflective of current family themes. These themes do not deal directly with the issues of affectional preference but rather the manner in which the family interacts with those persons inside and outside of the family unit. Some central themes that have impact on affectional preference issues and become barriers to dealing with the focal member in an open and supportive manner are "maintain respectibility at all costs," "be as our religion teaches us to be" and "as a family we can solve our own problems."

It is important that the practitioner gain a sense of how these elements present themselves in the system as a means for both predicting probable outcomes from strategic interventions and as a means for planning.

As the family system responds to inputs of affectional preference it appears to do so in five definable developmental stages. The interactions and transactions in the first three stages are with few exceptions characterized by adaptive systemic modes of denial.

The first response of the family system, *subliminal awareness,* generates a variety of homeostatic interactions with the focal member. These interactions manifest themselves as covert denial and control. Questions that might evoke a threatening response are not asked. Topics for conversation that might bring to light the issue are avoided. Interactions are always in such a manner so that the thrust of the interactions will be toward a maintenance of system functions as status quo. Parents often report that they sensed early in the child's development that same-gender orientation was present. They noted that behaviors of the focal member made them question sexual orientation but that fear of positive feedback hindered asking for an affirmative response. Parents at this point ask instead for behavioral responses that provide negative opportunities to deny the same-gender orientation. This pattern of interaction may be continued over a period of years at high cost to the system until overt behavior finally brings to clarity the existence of an affectional preference orientation and thus necessitates an immediate response. Disclosure then becomes the input of initial intervention. This input can be either gradual or abrupt, and as either direct input from the focal member or as a series of inputs from outside of the system. Questions raised by family friends, neighbors or family members concerning the lifestyle of the focal member or direct knowledge about the lifestyle of the focal member often contribute to the process of disclosure. The most disruptive input from outside of the system is a stigmatized disclosure in the form of an arrest for sexual misconduct.

In the family system where enmeshment and rigidity are present to a high degree disclosure by the gay man or lesbian may not take place for years unless forced from outside of the system. The focal member adopts a caretaking posture in reference to the family unit. Interactions with the family unit is in the form of highly ritualized social interchange. In addition many times the focal member will maintain a geographical distance from family members or at the extreme place himself or herself in self-exile.

Chaotic and disengaged systems often do not undergo the adaptive process as overt disclosure of affectional preference usually is not undertaken by the focal member. Gay men and lesbians whose family of origin are characterized by this type of constellation do not often feel a personal need to disclose their orientational preference as a means of reducing the personal stresses generated by the system. Interaction with the family system is not stressful because members in the family configuration do not connect with each other with an appreciable degree of affect or expectation. The focal member can easily lead a double existence especially if he or she continues to reside at a safe geographical distance from the family and maintains familial contact in a ritualized manner such as by letters, telephone calls and occasional family visits.

This stage of the family's development with respect to the issue generates guilt, a sense of isolation and anger within the focal member. He or she is needing family approval for himself or herself as a person but is threatened by the fear of rejection. The accumulated anger with a focus toward the family members is blocked by the system and refocused upon the focal member. It is important that this anger be confronted by the practitioner who is working with the individual focal member. This anger often masquerades as lowered self-esteem and depressive reactions. The most useful intervention is to assist the individual in the development of a disclosure procedure and a means for dealing with the outcomes of disclosure to the family.

When the system inputs have clarified the existence of a family member with a same-gender affectional preference orientation the family moves into the second stage, *impact*. This is the crisis stage and the stage at which most practitioners will make initial contact with the family. Rapid disorganization and system loss are present. Fear, guilt, perceived role failure and loss of boundaries are the central issues for the family. The sense of loss of control evokes responses that will maintain the idealized family fantasy. Active denial being a typical response. References are made to past behaviors that validate appropriate sex-role activity. In this response family members are unwilling to make clear the boundary between sex-role activity and sexual orientation. Inability to set this boundary keeps the family in a state of confusion which is the focal feeling for family members in this stage. There is a consensus among family members that this knowledge has dramatically affected them and they actively explore ways to deal with the resultant stress. The immediate request of the family is to remove the stress by removing the stressor, the focal member. This request is granted by the focal member by the distancing process of lessened contact to relieve stress and purchase time for the family.

The third stage *adjustment* occurs immediately following impact. The system must begin to restabilize in some manner. Reestablishment involves both external and internal coping mechanisms. Change in sexual orientation is first requested. When system inputs indicate that a change is not possible the family moves to a bargaining position with the focal member. He or she is asked to make concessions in lifestyle that will maintain the family's sense of respectability. The thrust is to manage the sexual orientation by regulative structures. Rules that will regulate the focal member's behavior are established. The spoken or unspoken rule becomes that of "keep your orientation a secret." The boundaries for this rule are usually external but in many families it is also internal.

Seldom is the knowledge of sexual preference disclosed to the family system as a whole but rather incrementally to selected family members. The first disclosure is made to the family member with whom the focal member has the strongest bond. It is not uncommon for this member to request a contract of secrecy. This sets boundaries for the management of the secret so that other family members are protected. The focal member who accepts this contract must generate separate sets of communication boundaries specific to each family member. This leads to confusion within the system, perceived structural chaos and double-binding relationships.

The mandate from the system is that the focal member actualize his or her orientation in such a way that his or her interactions do little if any damage to the family's image or disturb drastically other family themes. For example, the family where religious teachings are internalized as major family themes will experience aggravated stress in its dealings with affectional preference issues. This stress causes the system to utilize religious practice and teachings as a means of controlling the focal member. One family with whom I worked recounted the use of daily prayer sessions as a means of strengthening the guilt response in the focal member and garnering control over her lesbian lifestyle.

The tendency for the family system at this stage is to focus on actions rather than on feelings. When the actions of the focal member comply with the requests of the system the process is brought to a temporary closure with unresolved anger. The family falsely believe that it has resolved the issues relative to affectional preference. It is at this point that many families will remove themselves from therapeutic intervention unless the practitioner calls for the resolution of the residual feelings.

The key to this resolution is an understanding that control may alleviate stress and create a sense of family well-being but that only when the system acknowledges the impact of the affectional preference and can deal with its presence in an open, honest and forthright manner without control over the focal member's lifestyle will true resolution come to fruition. This understanding can be given to the family members if the practitioner continually confronts the real issues, clarifies the interactions that are taking place and requests feelings.

If the family can develop the understanding and open the system it can move to the *resolution* phase. This phase affords the family the opportunity to combine feelings with its perceived sense of losses and to mourn the demise of the focal family member. It is absolutely necessary that the practitioner foster this sense of loss. The work of the family at this stage is to readjust family rules, roles and themes. Knowledge is critical to the completion of this stage. The knowledge need be affirmative in nature so that it eradicates negative stereotypes projecting a sense of worth for the focal member. The family with this knowledge can actively confront the myths that have been internalized from the social environment. Active confrontation negates the fears that same-gender sexual orientation is sick, sinful and shameful.

In working with families in this stage I employ a grief and loss approach with input of affirmative knowledge. Little by little, I confront the stereotypes held by the family and replace them with positive images of the gay and lesbian lifestyle. I assist the family in expressing the losses that they will experience with a family member with same-gender orientation. These losses vary from family to family. For some families marriage and potential for childbirth may be a loss and for other families it is not. It is not important that I can identify for the family the losses but rather that I guide the family through a series of potential losses and help them validate them. My demand in working with families is for openness at all levels and mutual support. Teaching the family how to maintain an open system is central to my intervention.

Having mourned the loss of family expectations, gained affirmative knowledges, dispelled negative myths and confronted its fears the family can now move into the final stage *integration*. The family will remain in this stage during the lifetime of the focal member.

Throughout its tenure in this stage the family will continuously change its structure to accommodate the lifecycle movements of the focal member. With the skills gained in the previous stage the family has the capacity to promote self-actualization characterized by open communication and acceptance. Initial movements in this manner will be difficult for the family but facility will be gained with each new encounter. As one mother stated to my parent support group, "Just when we think everything is resolved our son's gayness again becomes central to our family. But, then, no more so than does his sister's heterosexuality."

INTERVENTION STRATEGY

When one selects to work with families where affectional preference is an issue the role undertaken is that of guide. The worker utilizes techniques that assist the family members through the crisis of unmet expectations and broken rules when no rules exist for current behavior, no role fit exists for the focal member, no constructive language exists to facilitate coping with the situation and strong family and cultural sanctions exist against the behavior. Successful therapeutic intervention is abortive when the practitioner holds personal negative value assumptions, utilizes stigmatizing clinical labels or paradigms, or is unclear about personal feeling relative to affectional preference minorities.

As is the case with most successful therapeutic interventions the success level is higher when there exists a "fit" with the family system. For the practitioner this requires the undertaking of a careful assessment of the dynamics of the family system. This assessment necessitates gaining an understanding of how the family interacts around issues not related to the issue of affectional preference. The assessment further includes gaining a sense of the real issues evoked by the affectional preference orientation of the focal member as family members often are unable to identify the true source of their discomfort. The practitioner can facilitate the family's inspection of each family member's issues in relationship to his or her interaction with the focal member. It is important to focus upon the feelings evoked by the interaction with the focal member. It is the feelings concerning the issues that will define the relationship's course for the future.

In working with families with affectional preference as an issue I have found the following intervention behaviors on my part to be useful in assisting the families confront the issue: Confront the individuals when feelings are not expressed. When feelings are expressed, validate them. Clarify responses that are homophobic in nature. Confront denial whenever it occurs. Be cognizant of the system's potential for punishment. Confront efforts to scapegoat the focal member. Clarify attempts to maintain idealized family fantasy. Be specific, concrete and explicit when contracting with family members. Affirm alternative organizational rules for the family when they open up the system. Speak the unspoken rules. Assist in redefinition of family roles. Articulate personal biases. Last, avoid encouraging adjustment. Instead, strive for resolution.

RESOURCES FOR THE PRACTITIONER

These intervention behaviors alone will not bring about successful therapeutic intervention if the practitioner comes to the therapy without a personal sense of affirmation for a same-gender affectional preference orientation and a collection of affirmative resources.

For practitioners who are not knowledgeable about gay and lesbian issues and are seeking an affirmative set of readings, I direct them to the Board of Social and Ethical Responsibility for Psychology Committee on Gay Concerns' *A Selected Bibliography of Gay Concerns in Psychology: An Affirmative Perspective,* Washington, D.C: American Psychological Association, August, 1982. This bibliography includes a wide spectrum of gay and lesbian issues for background reading as well as specific references useful to family members.

The isolation felt by the family members as they deal with the issues often can be lessened if the practitioner can connect the family with a support group. A national affiliation of these groups exists in the P-FLAG, Parents-Friends of Lesbians and Gays, organization. Not all cities have chapters but the list of newly formed chapters is continually expanding. The focus of the group is on education and a sharing of common experience with emphasis upon the development of family solidarity. A listing of the chapters may be secured by writing the organization at P.O. Box 24565, Los Angeles, California 90024.

Meeting the Needs
of Sexual Minority Youth:
One Program's Response

Tacie L. Vergara

ABSTRACT. This article brings the needs of sexual minority youth to the attention of the social work profession. The author describes the experiences of the Eromin Center, Inc. in developing a comprehensive youth services program to meet the special needs of sexual minority youth and provides practical guidelines for social workers who wish to work effectively with this population.

INTRODUCTION

As Dulaney and Kelly (1982) have stated in a recent issue of *Social Work,* "Despite the now well documented fact that 10% of the population in the United States of America is homosexual, the social work profession too often acts as though this significant minority is unworthy of serious consideration" (p. 178). An important subgroup of this minority has received even less attention. Virtually nothing has been done by social workers to address the needs of the severely oppressed, invisible and outcast adolescent sexual minority population. This article attempts to bring the issues of sexual minority youth out of the closet and to the attention of the social work profession and into the social service agency.

After a brief discussion concerning language, often a source of confusion and misinformation, an overview is provided so that helping professionals can recognize sexual minority youth and their special needs. The majority of this article is devoted to a dis-

A debt of thanks is owed to Anthony Silvestre, the Executive Director of Eromin Center, Inc. and to Mary Cochran, the Clinical Director of the Center and the Board of Directors. Their vision, leadership and dedication to sexual minorities have been key ingredients in developing the Youth Service Program.

19

cussion of developing services to meet the needs of sexual minority youth from individual, agency and institutional perspectives. At the conclusion, specific guidelines for social workers who wish to respond to and meet the needs of sexual minority youth are provided.

THE IMPORTANCE OF LANGUAGE

Language is a vehicle of communication; it also has political and psychological importance in that it significantly affects how we think about ourselves and others. Throughout the body of this article, the terms sexual minority youth, gay youth, and homosexual youth will be used interchangeably. While it is true that all gay youth are members of a sexual minority, not all sexual minority persons are gay. A sexual minority person may identify as homosexual, gay, lesbian, bisexual, transsexual or transvestite. The Eromin Center, Inc. program for sexual minority youth (which is the central focus of this article) serves primarily a gay population. However, a small percentage of the youth it serves identify as lesbian, bisexual or transsexual.

The Eromin Center, Inc. has historically served many sexual minorities (not just gay men and lesbians). Its commitment to continue to do so is reflected in the agency's staffing patterns, training plans and program descriptions. Hence there is also a commitment in the Youth Service Program to make services available to all sexual minority youth and not just gay and lesbian youth.

"Sexual Minority" is a relatively new term which has evolved largely to expand the current civil rights efforts beyond the particular issues of homosexuality. According to the Pennsylvania Council for Sexual Minorities, "the term 'sexual minority' is meant to encompass anyone whose romantic attachments or sexual behavior (either primary, as in actual sexual experience or secondary, as in clothing) is not dangerous to other people but significantly different from what we assume to be the norm" (Pennsylvania Department of Education, 1980, p. 4). Under the umbrella term "sexual minority," all other words which are used in defining and describing this population are subsumed. The Eromin Center, Inc., defines sexual minorities to include gay men, lesbians, bisexual, transvestites and transsexuals.

Until recently, the most common term used to define sexual minorities has been homosexual. Homosexual is a word which is used to define persons who relate sexually to other persons of their own gender.

"Gay" is currently a popular alternative to the word "homosexual," primarily because it is "our" word. It is common for oppressed persons, such as homosexuals, to claim their own words to define themselves and to communicate among themselves with pride. The word "gay" emerged as a way for homosexuals to communicate among and about themselves with pride. The word "gay" can be used to refer to persons, places and things such as gay restaurants, a gay fundraiser, or a gay friend. It is also appropriate to use the word "gay" when referring to both men and women. However, most people have used the words "gay" and "homosexual" to refer to men only. Therefore, many gay women prefer to think of themselves and to be referred to as "lesbians." The word "lesbian" has a "herstorical" association with a Greek Island, Lesbos, where a group of women lived together nearly 3,000 years ago. The word "lesbian," like the word "gay," has positive connotations. These are words that have pride associated with them, words that sexual minority youth need to learn.

Beyond language confusion, often other kinds of sexual behavior are confused with homosexuality (e.g., transvestism, transsexuality and bisexuality). Transvestites are men or women who "cross-dress" (i.e., wear clothing usually worn by persons of the opposite gender). What most people do not know about transvestites is that they are most often heterosexual, married men who "cross-dress" in the privacy of their own homes, for sexual or psychological gratification. There are some gay male transvestites who "cross-dress" in public; this is referred to as "being in drag" and these men are often called "drag queens." Transvestites are not to be confused with female impersonators. Female impersonators are men who earn their living "cross-dressing," performing in nightclubs. These men may be gay, heterosexual, or bisexual.

Transsexuals are persons who report feeling trapped in the wrong body. They are not persons who identify themselves as gay; in fact, this is rarely the case. Rather, these people psychologically identify themselves with the opposite biological gender and desire to be a person of that gender. Many transsexuals will eventually opt for sex reassignment surgery. Christine Jorgenson is a well-known example of a person who underwent this type of surgery. In many major cities in the United States, there are clinical programs for sex reassignment surgery which provide medically supervised pre-operative, operative and post-operative procedures. Prior to sex reassignment surgery, transsexuals may be attracted to persons of their biological gender; however, they do not experience these as gay attractions. Rather, they experience these as heterosexual attractions.

Bisexual is another word heard in discussions of sexual minorities. The term bisexual, appropriately used, refers to persons who identify neither exclusively as heterosexual nor exclusively as homosexual. They are attracted to people of the same sex and to people of the opposite sex.

Sexual minority youth are often confused by inappropriate labels that are used to define their sexual and affectional feelings. At least 50% of the gay male adolescent population that the Eromin Center staff saw on admission identified themselves as transsexual based solely on their sexual and affectional feelings toward men. Initial social work intervention with these gay adolescents was aimed at providing them with accurate information about this term. Additionally they were afforded an opportunity to explore their sexual and affectional feelings in a safe and supportive environment, with sensitive and informed persons. Within a relatively short period of time almost all of these youth were self-identifying as "gay." Sexual minority youth have little access to information, resources, or persons who can provide positive and accurate frames of reference regarding their sexual identity issues. Educating ourselves and others about the appropriate meanings of words used to define sexual minorities are essential first steps toward working effectively with this population. Communicating with sexual minority youth in language that is accurate and positive (e.g., that refers to homosexuality within the range of human sexuality) is vital. Language, our primary vehicle of communication, impacts directly on the development of self-image and self-esteem.

RECOGNIZING SEXUAL MINORITY YOUTH AND THEIR NEEDS: AN OVERVIEW

Sexual minority youth are often the most invisible subgroup of adolescents. Although the present prevailing view among social scientists is that gender identity and erotic preference are established very early in life, most helping professionals continue to perpetuate the myth that young men and women cannot be sure of their sexual preference (Myths and Stereotypes, Note 1).

Overlooking the reality that sexual minority youth exist and need services has serious repercussions. Sexual minority youth may commit suicide, deny or repress the sexual dimension of their identity, or feel alone, frightened and alienated in a homophobic society (Lenna and Woodman, 1981, p. 1). If, on the other hand, sexual minority youth refuse to accept the invisible status assigned them by society, they are often subject to ridicule, hostility and rejection.

The cumulative effects of being either an invisible or outcast segment of society are often that sexual minority youth feel bad about themselves, have a poor self-image and low self-esteem, and more than other teenagers, feel totally alone. Many gay youth run away and become involved in prostitution and drug trafficking. Homeless gay youth, living on the streets in major cities, are subject to physical and sexual abuse by disturbed and violent people. The staff at Huckleberry House, a short-term residential program for young people ages 12-17 in San Francisco, report that gay youth have higher incidences of suicide attempts, that these youth report a higher rate of physical abuse at home, and that they drop out of school more frequently than other clients because of harassment, ridicule and fear of physical attacks (Gibson, 1982).

Young people who are members of sexual minorities or who are confused about their sexual orientation or sexual minority status (or that of their parents) often find it difficult to deal successfully with their situations. These young people often become confused by the negative reactions of their parents, peers, social service workers, teachers and foster parents resulting in increased isolation, insecurity and acting-out behavior.

Families with these young people, especially if dealing with other problems (and many of them are), find sexual minority issues greatly compound their difficulties. Placement of sexual minority youth in traditional foster homes often creates problems, since untrained foster parents are rarely more successful in understanding sexual minority issues than the general population. It has been clearly shown in the United States and Canada that placing sexual minority youth in nonsensitive heterosexual foster families and group homes repeats the original family dynamic and leads to placement failure (Saperstein, 1981, p. 61). Children placed in these homes often find barriers to communication and successful functioning.

Placement of sexual minority youth in institutions is rarely successful since some staff members deny the presence of sexual minority youth and most staff members are not trained to deal with them. Too often, these adolescents are sexually victimized by their peers. Prior to being placed with Eromin, one of our residents had been repeatedly gang raped while in residential care. On one occasion, the sexual abuse was coupled with severe physical abuse. The severity of the physical abuse led to this youngster's being removed from placement. He was then temporarily placed in foster care with his sister where he was again sexually and physically abused, this time by his sister's male lover. This history of sexual and physical abuse is not an unusual occurrence. At least 50% of the residents in Eromin's group home program have had similar sexual and physical abuse experiences while in placements.

Although sexual minority youth represent a significant population group (Gibson, Note 2), these young people have few advocates and virtually no power or authority to demand the provision and/or improvement of social services to meet their specific needs. It is social workers who must advocate for these youth. In order to do this, social workers must first recognize that sexual minority youth exist and need services. Social workers and other professionals in the human services field must then acknowledge that sexual minority youth are found everywhere services are provided, such as in programs serving children in their own homes, outpatient mental health clinics, inpatient psychiatric facilities, juvenile detention centers, foster homes, short and long-term residential treatment facilities, runaway and other emergency shelters, schools and residential programs such as group homes. Sexual minority youth are adjudicated dependent, delinquent and committed to psychiatric inpatient facilities. They are also youth who walk into voluntary agencies. They are youth who want and need our help.

THE EROMIN CENTER YOUTH SERVICES PROGRAM

History

In order to meet the needs of sexual minority youth, we must first identify this "invisible population" and then advocate for services to meet their stated needs. Two social workers from the Philadelphia Department of Public Welfare's Children and Youth Program did just that. In 1979, Russell Cardamone and John Sahner began to advocate for the needs of sexual minority youth. Armed with the 1977 National Association of Social Workers (NASW) Delegate Assembly Policy Statement (NASW, Note 3), the NASW Code of Ethics (NASW, Note 4), and their position paper indicating the potential numbers of gay and lesbian youth who were not being served, these two men requested a meeting with the Director of the Philadelphia County Children and Youth Agency. As a result of this meeting, a study committee on sexual minority issues was formed. Six committee members were appointed and charged with the responsibility of studying the issues regarding the provision of services to sexual minorities and to make recommendations. A research coordinator was assigned to survey the caseloads of social workers to determine the number of sexual minority youth who were in the care of Philadelphia County's Children and Youth Agency.

At the time this survey was conducted, no one had received training in identifying gay and lesbian youth. However, 49 lesbian and gay youth were identified. It is interesting to note that only 21 social workers, out of a possible 200–300, responded to this survey. Of the 49 identified, 29 of these youth were in placement and 20 were receiving non-placement services. It was further ascertained from this survey, that six of the 29 youth in placement could have been returned home immediately if there were support services for the families to deal with sexual minority issues. Further, 53% of the respondents in the survey indicated a strong desire for training in dealing with sexual minority youth. The study committee on sexual minority issues compiled a report indicating its findings and recommended priority be given to staff training, counseling and intervention services, and a foster care program to meet the needs of sexual minority youth.

At the request of the Department of Public Welfare, Eromin Center (through Temple University) offered three separate one and one-half day workshops in March, April and May of 1980. These workshops focused specifically on sexual minority issues. Ninety-five percent of the social workers from the Philadelphia County Children and Youth Agency participated in the training. Trainees received 1.4 Continuing Education Units and the training was funded by Title XX. The training focused on: attitudes on working with sexual minority persons; values clarification; social and psychological research data regarding these minorities; and issues in working with sexual minorities in accordance with agency policies and goals. The impact of this training was threefold; (1) increasing numbers of sexual minority youth were identified; (2) some social workers at all three workshops identified themselves as either gay or lesbian; and (3) there was a groundswell of support from Philadelphia County Children and Youth social workers for a foster care program for sexual minority youth. This information was brought to the Director and, on June 16, 1980, he wrote to Anthony Silvestre, the Executive Director of Eromin Center, Inc., to request the development of foster care and non-placement counseling services for sexual minority youth. The Eromin Center, Inc. began providing foster care for sexual minority youth on September 1, 1980.

The efforts of Cardamone and Sahner were clearly directed toward operationalizing social work practice objectives (e.g., helping people enlarge their competence and increase their problem-solving and coping abilities, helping people obtain resources, influencing interactions between organizations and institutions, influencing policy, and not discriminating on the basis of sexual orientation) (Social Work, 1981, p. 6).

The Context

The Eromin Center, Inc. was founded in 1973 as the only non-profit, professional counseling and educational center in Eastern Pennsylvania for sexual minorities. The agency was developed in response to the need for non-prejudicial mental health services to members of sexual minorities. Since 1973, the Eromin Center has pioneered in providing human services to the sexual minority community and has grown considerably in size and scope. The current range of services available includes information and referral, counseling (individual, group, couples, and family), community education and training programs, and, most recently, a comprehensive youth service program.

Licensed by the Commonwealth of Pennsylvania both as an outpatient psychiatric clinic and as a children and youth agency, The Eromin Center is recognized as a major source of information and referral by federal, state and local governments, national, state and local sexual minority organizations and by public and private businesses and foundations. Eromin's revenues are generated through client fees, third-party providers, grants, government contracts, private contributions, donations and fund-raising efforts. Community volunteers provide over $250,000 of in-kind services each year. The Eromin Center is committed to improving and developing services so that every sexual minority person can count on help when it is needed (Eromin Center, Inc., 1981).

The Youth Service Program

Eromin Center's Youth Service Program works almost exclusively with a black, male, adolescent, sexual minority population. The sexual minority youth in Eromin's Youth Program all have long histories of involvement with children and youth agencies; most of the program's population is adjudicated dependent. Psychosocial summaries almost invariably reflect backgrounds which include physical and sexual abuse, emotional neglect, and early developmental years characterized by harsh treatment, a lack of consistent parenting, and frequent transitory living situations in inadequate dwellings.

At least 50% of the male adolescents served have been involved in juvenile prostitution. Also, approximately 50% have been sexually abused while in placements provided by County Children and Youth Agencies and supervised by human service professionals. Additionally, 25% of the population have been runaways or throwaways: these young men run away from placements where they are not protected or they are thrown out of families who refuse to view their sexual minority status as anything but sick.

Counseling and Outreach Services. Prior to developing a specific program for sexual minority youth, Eromin had been providing outreach and counseling services to adolescents since 1973. The continued provision of this vital service has kept the agency in touch with the many and varied needs of sexual minority youth. Typically, adolescents do not have the money to pay for these services and they are therefore made available at little or no cost.

Foster Home Care. Sexual minority youth in need of foster care placements have typically experienced significant conflict in their natural home or another foster care situation. The Eromin Center foster care program provides sexual minority youth with an accepting home environment, a safe living situation, and contact with nonexploitative gay or gay-sensitive adults to supervise and guide them to mature and productive life styles. The goals of foster care placement vary according to the needs of the youth and their families. Emergency short-term care is provided for some

youth until the youth and their natural family have the time and resources to work out the problems which led to placement. Temporary short-term foster care is provided for youth who are preparing
for independent living and who, for whatever reasons, cannot return home. Long-term foster care is provided for youth until they
are eighteen if they cannot be returned home.

Identifying gay and gay-sensitive foster parents to meet the
needs of sexual minority youth is a challenge. Gay and gay-sensitive foster parents are not an already existing, visible segment of
society. Therefore, typical recruitment efforts such as press releases, newspaper ads, flyers, posters, speaking engagements, etc.
cannot be relied upon to reach this group. Since we assume that
sexual minority persons are everywhere, our recruiting efforts are
not limited to gay publications or organizations. Rather, we appeal
to the community at large when we are recruiting foster parents.
We have learned, as have many other agencies which provide foster care for a special population, that the most effective recruiting
efforts come from both personal contacts and word-of-mouth referrals. There are some special considerations we address in screening and approving foster care applicants. Eromin actively recruits
foster parents who are interested in and capable of being role models for sexual minority youth and who can prepare these youth for
independent living, as most sexual minority youth in need of
placement do not return home but rather go on to live on their own
(Gibson, Note 5).

In recruiting foster parent applicants, Eromin gives priority to
gay adults. Gay youth have too few positive role models with
which to identify; our foster parents fulfill this need if they are
comfortable with their own sexual minority status in their communities, their workplaces, and their family and friendship networks.
An assessment of their comfort level with their own sexual minority status is made in the initial screening process. We prefer gay
foster homes for sexual minority youth because we assume that
there will be a higher degree of acceptance and understanding for
the special needs of these youth and hence a higher degree of success for both the youth and the foster parents.

Eromin faces the issue of sexual exploitation of youth neither
more nor less than any other agency. Therefore, in identifying
homes for our youth, we are direct and specific about this concern
and the agency's policy. Eromin explicitly states that persons acting in the capacity of adult caretakers are forbidden to have sexual

contact with the youth in their care under any circumstances. Further, we consider sexual activity between youths and their adult caretakers sexually exploitative acts and will decertify foster homes and assist youths in prosecuting if necessary. Originally, the Eromin staff thought that, in order to protect against the sexual exploitation of our youth, we should put a great deal of time and effort into identifying gay couples who have been in long-standing, stable relationships. For a variety of reasons, finding such gay male couples willing to serve as foster parents was difficult. Partly because these couples were not found and partly as a result of re-thinking our own image about who can be the "best" parent/guardians, we began to identify, screen and approve both single gay male and single gay-sensitive male foster parents. We have had considerable success with these placements. We have had less success in placing sexual minority youth in the homes of lesbian couples and in the homes of single lesbians. This may be unique to our population; it is too early to be definitive. This phenomenon is worth watching over time in our program and in other programs around the country.

Once foster homes are approved, it is essential that the Agency provide foster parents with on-going training. In addition to the foster parent training required by the state, Eromin provides special training programs to foster parents to help them meet the special needs of youth in their care. Special training is provided regarding sex role stereotyping and "coming out" issues for sexual minority youth, health issues (including sexually transmitted diseases), and identifying gay and gay-sensitive resources and support networks for both the foster parents and the youth.

Unlike their heterosexual counterparts, homosexual foster parents have few, if any, natural sources of support. Therefore, Eromin needs to provide ongoing support for their foster parents, and assists them in developing their own networks. Additionally, Eromin provides respite care for youth when foster parents need to be away (e.g., business, a death in the family, a vacation alone or with friends). Eromin also provides youth and foster parents the opportunity to be involved in social and recreational activities which include both the staff and other sexual minority youth in Eromin's program.

Group Home Care. In October, 1980, the Immigration and Naturalization Service asked the Eromin Center to develop services for a number of Cuban refugee youth, housed at Fort Indiantown

Gap, who had been identified as sexual minorities. These young men had been raped and abused. In addition to their immediate needs for counseling and shelter, these young men also needed intensive skills training. A staff, almost completely bilingual, was hired to provide counseling, recreation and residential services. Eromin Center's group home was named Eromin House. The young Cuban men, ranging in age from 16 to 18, were prepared for independent living or sponsorship at Eromin House. In May, 1981, Eromin House began accepting referrals from the Philadelphia Department of Public Welfare for sexual minority youth who needed group home services. Since then, Delaware County (PA), Northampton County (PA), and the State of New Jersey also have requested group home services.

Adolescents requiring residential care have typically experienced conflicts in other areas of their life (home, school, community and friendship networks). Their needs are broad and often independent of sexual or affectional preference. Eromin House has developed a four-pronged program which addresses the residential, educational, counseling and recreational needs of youth. The program is fully coordinated and totally focused on preparation of youth for successful independent living. The ultimate goals are to assist youths in meeting their individual objectives and to help them define sexual identities which are personally satisfying.

The *residential* needs of group home residents are met by providing them a safe, supportive, structured and accepting environment in which to live. The group home is staffed by human service professionals of various sexual orientations who provide the youth positive role models in non-sexual situations. The provision of such role models is essential to the development of positive self-images. In providing residential care for sexual minority youth, a challenge is to keep a balance between issues of sex and sexuality and other important issues. For instance, like other residential settings for adolescents, Eromin House has policies which attempt to regulate sexual activity in the house. However, unlike other programs, we are not overly concerned about a violation of this policy (neither more nor less than we are concerned about transgressions of other house rules). Certainly, we are not outraged by sexual activity between same-sex persons. It is important to note that it is not the act of sex that we are objecting to, hence residential counselors are cautioned not to label the acts or feelings as bad. However, since peaceful coexistence in group homes is facilitated by relating to each other as "family," residents are counseled to identify other sexual outlets that are acceptable in the house, such as masturbation. Validation of the feelings of how difficult it is to be an adolescent in this society, particularly in the area of expression of sexuality, is an important ingredient in the discussion following an incident of sexual activity in the house. This discussion must also include a touch of reality (i.e., there will always be rules of conduct that people must comply with in order to coexist peacefully with each other; some of these rules will be uncomfortable for people but they will need to be followed anyway).

The *educational* needs of our youth are met both in the community and by the provision of a licensed in-house educational program. A large percentage of our youth have been subjected to verbal and physical abuse and harassment in the public school system. This abuse and harassment has often led to avoidance of school or disruptive behavior which has caused innumerable suspensions and expulsions. The final results are severe educational handicaps (50% of our in-house school population, ages 16 to 17½, read at a second to fourth grade level) and strongly negative feelings about school and learning (at least 25% of our in-house school population are extremely school phobic). Our in-house school program was designed to provide individual learning programs and one-to-one attention and tutoring provided by trained educators and volunteers. In addition to teaching the basic subjects covered in all schools, our educators use special materials to provide a gay-sensitive curriculum. As Dr. Billy S. Jones noted in "The Needs for Cultural Sensitivity in Working with Third World Lesbian and Gay Youth," "When one part of yourself is secret, that becomes the most important part of you" (Jones, 1982). For the youth in our educational program being a sexual minority is no longer a secret, unlike their experience in public schools. It is our view that being able to attach equal importance to all parts of themselves frees sexual minority youth up to devote needed attention to their educational growth and development.

The *counseling* needs of the youth at Eromin House are met in two ways. Each youth is given an individual residential counselor to review with them their overall progress in the program and to help them overcome obstacles to maximum functioning in the group home setting. Secondly, the counseling needs of our youth are met by matching them with individual therapists whom they see on a weekly basis. While most group homes provide youths with residential counselors, few require that youths be involved in ongoing psychotherapy. We provide this service for several reasons. First, most of our youth have been in sexually, physically and emotionally abusive relationships with adult caretakers; hence they fear closeness and intimacy and lack trust. Secondly, often youths who have been thrown out of their families are faced with guilt and self-doubt. Finally, we welcome additional opportunities to provide role models who can facilitate the development of positive self-images in our youth.

The *recreational* needs of our youth are met through the collaboration of the residential counselor/activities specialist, school personnel, and interested youth, who develop a monthly activities schedule. Our population are less interested than most youths in group homes in combative, competitive, and aggressive games; nor are they interested in team sports. This may be due to the association of these activities with heterosexual males, to fear of competition due to underdeveloped self images, or to a combination of these and other factors. The recreational activities we have found to be successful with our population include more solitary endeavors such as dance, body-building, painting, and creative writing workshops (poetry and journal writing). Concerts and theatre are good choices for group ventures. House games based on luck as opposed to skill, movies, and arts and crafts activities are also popular. It is important that we choose games that are not sex-role stereotyped or highly competitive, that we offer a range of options, and that we invite the residents to participate in planning individual and group recreational activities.

Service to Children in their Own Homes (SCOH). While we see Group Home Care and Foster Care as two essential program components for sexual minority youth (and we have many more requests for service than we can fill), Eromin Center is committed to the belief that the natural family is crucial to child rearing and that the family must be preserved whenever possible. Eromin is committed to encouraging youth to maintain contact and communication with their families and to working with the natural parents whenever possible. One of our service goals is returning youths to their home as soon as possible. The provision of Services to Children in their Own Homes (SCOH) reflects this philosophy. However, it is important to note that these are the most underutilized services in the Eromin Youth Program. We believe that there are several reasons for this. First, SCOH clients come to our attention much later than SCOH clients in most other programs. Further-more, removal of a sexual minority youth from the natural home often seems like the only tolerable option to a family which ac-cepts myths and stereotypes about homosexuality. Some special considerations in providing SCOH services are worth mentioning. Again, it is important to have counselors/therapists of various sex-ual orientations. In family therapy, it is optimal to have a homo-sexual and heterosexual counseling team in order for the sexual minority person and other family members to have someone with whom they can identify as issues involving sexuality are explored in family therapy sessions. In working with families it is important to keep a balance between the sexual orientation issue and other is-sues. In working with families, it is advisable to watch for other problems which may be masquerading as "one of the family mem-bers is gay." It is not unusual for the gay-identified client to be scapegoated (Wirth, 1982). Connecting the family with resources such as Parents and Friends of Gays (About Our Children, 1982) and other support networks may assist them in accepting their child's sexual minority status. Gay youth groups may help the sex-ual minority youth understand the process their parents are going through and provide sexual minority youth the support that they temporarily cannot get from their family. Facilitating acceptance on both sides may encourage reunion between sexual minority youth and their families.

Supervised Independent Living. Sexual minority youth are often forced out of their homes or leave unprepared for the realities of living on their own. Without high school diplomas, employment skills, and stable residency records, these youths face major obsta-cles in obtaining housing and employment. It is not unusual for these youths to exchange their bodies for food, clothing and shel-ter. Supervised Independent Living will assist us in placing youth in individual rental apartments or in boarding home settings in the community together with social work supervision and supportive services. We will be able to provide the long-term financial, emo-tional, educational and vocational support needed to help these sexual minority youth lead healthy and productive lives. This pro-gram is in its developmental stages: constructing various forms and assessment tools, identifying Life Skills specialists, coordinating with the educational program to provide a life-skills curriculum for eligible candidates and developing and implementing policies and procedures specifically applicable to this program. Identifying gay-sensitive and youth-sensitive real estate agents is the first obstacle to overcome in housing these youth. Use of the gay community's informal network has proven to be our most valuable resource for identifying potential housing opportunities. It is important that youth who are candidates for this program participate in a preparatory program to identify gay or gay-sensitive medical, legal, social, religious, and other community resources. Special attention must be given to employment opportunities, especially since sexual minority youth are in double or triple jeopardy for unemployment.

It is our hope that youth involved in Eromin's supervised independent living program will be able, with our help, to overcome obstacles to housing, employment and other services, and that they will be able to gradually acquire the necessary life skills to manage the expectations and responsibilities of adulthood. The goal of this program is to ensure that sexual minority youth do not become "street gays" or systems-dependent adults. A six-month follow-up built into this program will help us to evaluate our success.

Service Philosophy. A philosophy about human sexuality flows through Eromin's Youth Services Programs: What really matters about sexuality is its incorporation within human relationships which are caring, responsible, loving and honest. We work toward the advancement of these attitudes rather than the development of one's sexual orientation. Sexuality is viewed as a function of the total personality and we understand the impact of sexuality on personality development, interpersonal relationships and, hence, on society. Eromin does not have a genital approach to services (i.e., we do not focus on with whom a person chooses to have an actual sexual relationship). Rather, we have a whole-person approach to service, are concerned with the psychosocial development of our youth, and place a heavy programmatic emphasis on responsibility for self, building self-esteem, and career development.

GUIDELINES AND SUGGESTIONS FOR OTHERS

The experience of the Eromin Center, Inc. can provide helpful principles and guidelines for those who are interested in providing needed services to sexual minority youth. If social workers are to be effective in their dealings with sexual minority youth, they must educate themselves about sexual minority issues and use sensitive terminology. An examination of the beliefs and assumptions held about sexual minorities is also essential. Almost everyone accepts some stereotypes about homosexuality. Erroneous and harmful messages about sexual minorities are transmitted through literature and the media. If erroneous beliefs and assumptions go unchallenged and unexamined by the social work profession, they will continue to stand between sexual minorities and effective services. In working with sexual minority youth, social workers should draw on basic social work tenets (e.g., starting where the client is and establishing an atmosphere of acceptance). These principles of the profession are especially important in working with sexual minority youth. Conveying an attitude of acceptance of difference can be accomplished in various ways. The types of questions we ask, how we respond (both verbally and non-verbally) and the types of books, magazines and pictures we have in the waiting room and in our offices are all important to consider.

At each stage in developing services to meet the needs of sexual minority youth, there are particular roadblocks and obstacles to be overcome. Identifying the population to be served is the first stage in developing any program; however in most youth programs there is a denial system about the existence of sexual minority youth. This is reflected in intake and admissions forms and procedures which do not concern themselves with a youth's sexual or affectional preference. A worker interested in identifying this "invisible" population could counteract this by keeping a statistical compilation sheet which identifies a case number (not name) and the sexual orientation and gender of the client. This sheet could also be used to document the special services that were needed but which the agency could not provide.

Once the population is identified and their needs for service are documented, the social worker has to advocate for these youth and their needs. Advocacy efforts include, among other things, bringing to the attention of program administrators the reality that sexual minority youth exist and need services that their agency is not providing. Further, social workers should insist that agencies enforce sexual orientation and non-discrimination policies where they exist and help develop such policies where they do not.

If the agency intends to develop services to meet the special needs of sexual minority youth, funding to provide staff training and to develop new and specialized services will be required. Obtaining funding will undoubtedly present a challenge. Public and private funding agencies do not look favorably on agencies which support behavior considered unacceptable by many. Sparky Harlan (1982), in her article, "Development and Administration of Lesbian and Gay Youth Services," suggests various ways of dealing with funding obstacles. For instance, Ms. Harlan suggests that using the wider category of sexual minority youth (which includes juvenile prostitutes and sexually abused youth) can assist in broadening funding opportunities and providing needed services. Incorporating gay youth services with other youth services whenever possible may have financial and programmatic benefits. Identifying funding sources which specifically fund unique and innovative programs is also recommended (Harlan, 1982). Other methods to overcome funding blocks include: identifying gay business-person associations and gay-sensitive service organizations (which can be found in most large metropolitan areas) for financial support, and using various formal and informal resources in the gay community to identify potential funding sources. Having a Board of Directors which is supportive of the services, understands the funding dilemmas incumbent in developing such services, and is committed to raising the funds necessary to provide specialized services is particularly advantageous.

CONCLUSION

An essential beginning step for social work practitioners, planners, and administrators in meeting the needs of sexual minority youth is to embrace the truth about this population: that sexual minority youth exist and need services that they do not receive. While the NASW and other professional organizations have made major policy statements declaring homosexuality a viable lifestyle devoid of psychopathology, little has been done to encourage the development of sensitive and effective services for sexual minorities, especially sexual minority youth. Social workers must move beyond educating themselves, examining their beliefs and assumptions, and writing policy statements that support the professional Code of Ethics. It is time to back up words with actions; with programs that are responsive to the needs of adult and adolescent sexual minority persons. Eromin Center Youth Services is an example of a program developed to meet the needs of a sexual minority youth population. There needs to be more programs like this around the country.

REFERENCE NOTES

1. Myths and Stereotypes. *Gay Youth Counseling Manual.* "According to prominent social scientists such as John Money and Lawrence Kohlberg, the sexual orientation of a child is established before the age of four." Unpublished Manual, National Network of Runaway and Youth Services, 1982.
2. Gibson, P. Developing Services to Gay and Lesbian Youth in a Runaway Shelter. Gibson reports that more than 55% of the clients at Huckleberry House are sexual minority youth. Sexual minority youth as defined by this program include Gay, Lesbian, and Bisexual youth, youth prostitutes and young people who have been sexually abused. Of these 55%, 25% identify themselves as Gay, Lesbian or Bisexuals. *Gay Youth Counseling Manual.* Unpublished Manual, National Network of Runaway and Youth Services, 1982.
3. *National Association of Social Workers Task Force on Gay Issues, An Introduction.* In 1977, the NASW Delegate Assembly adopted a policy statement which, for the first time in the history of the profession, not only encouraged but mandated that, "NSAW concern itself with the eradication of prejudice and discrimination against Lesbian and Gay men in such areas as social policy and programs within health and welfare agencies (e.g., police departments), laws proscribing "consensual" relationships in private, employment and personnel practices, academic research and court action related to child custody visitation." Washington, D.C.: National Association of Social Work, Inc.
4. *Code of Ethics of the National Association of Social Workers:* "the social worker should not practice, condone, facilitate or collaborate with any form of discrimination on the basis of race, color, sex, sexual orientation, age, religion, national origin, marital status, political beliefs, mental or physical handicap and other preference or personal characteristics, condition or status." Washington, D.C.: National Association of Social Workers, Inc., 1980.
5. Gibson, P. Developing Services to Gay and Lesbian Youth in a Runaway Shelter. Gibson reports that fewer than 10% of the Gay clients they see at Huckleberry House are reunited with their families: Family reunification is often not an option for them. *Gay Youth Counseling Manual.* Unpublished Manual, National Network of Runaway and Youth Services, 1982.

REFERENCES

About our children. Los Angeles, California: Federation of Parents and Friends of Gays, Inc., 1982.
Dulaney, D.D. and Kelly, J. Improving services to gay and lesbian clients. *Social Work,* 1982, 27(2), 178.
Eromin Center, Inc. Philadelphia, Pa.: Agency Brochure, 1981.
Gibson, P. Developing services to gay and lesbian youth in a runaway shelter. *Gay youth counseling manual.* Unpublished manual, National Network of Runaway and Youth Services, 1982.
Harlan, S. Development and administration of lesbian and gay youth services. *Gay Youth Counseling Manual.* Unpublished manual, National Network of Runaway and Youth Services, 1982.

Jones, B.A.S. The need for cultural sensitivity in working with third world lesbian and gay youth. *Gay Youth Counseling Manual*. Unpublished manual, National Network of Runaway and Youth Services, 1982.

Lenna, H.R. & Woodman, W.J. *Face up to reality: Lesbian and gay youth exist and often want help*. Unpublished paper, Arizona State University and the University of Delaware, 1981.

Saperstein, S. Lesbian and gay adolescents the need for family support. *Catalyst*, 1981, *3*(4), 61.

What is a sexual minority anyway? Harrisburg, Pa.: Pa. Department of Education, 1980, 4.

Wirth, S. Principles for psychotherapy with families of lesbians and gay men. *Gay Youth Counseling Manual*. Unpublished manual, National Network of Runaway and Youth Services, 1982.

Working statement of the purpose of social work. *Social Work*, 1981, *26*(1), 6.

Counseling Gay and Lesbian Couples

Beverly Decker

ABSTRACT. Although lesbians and gay men in relationships are part of the client population that social workers serve, the critical dynamic and cultural issues involved in providing optimal help for same-sex couples have received little attention in the profession. The author discusses some of the unique characteristics and special problems of same-sex dyads which must be taken into consideration when theoretical and clinical issues are combined to form an effective treatment approach. Topics addressed include: How problems in defining boundaries of same-sex couples are intensified by the absence of social "rules" relating to them, the effects of homophobia on issues of oneness and differentiation, and the impact of gender socialization on differences between gay male and lesbian relationships.

INTRODUCTION

Despite the now well-documented fact that up to 10 percent or more of the population is homosexual (Marmor, 1980), social work professionals have too often acted as though this significant minority did not exist. Where articles have focused on improving services to homosexual clients have appeared in the literature, the special problems of lesbian and gay male couples are often ignored (Dulaney & Kelly, 1982). Where serious consideration has been given to such couples, the result, as Toder (1979) points out, has often been to take either the politically radical position that gay couples don't or shouldn't have anything in common with non-gay couples, or the well-meaning liberal position that same-sex couples are just like other married couples and, therefore, require no special understanding.

Certainly, there are obvious ways in which same-sex couples struggle with many of the same issues as heterosexual couples. Gay couples go to work, plan vacations, pay bills, and deal with illness, aging parents, and the deaths of family and friends. Many of their relational problems can be traced to the same developmental issues and family scripts that cause problems for heterosexual couples. In gay and non-gay couples alike, conflicts can arise if the individuals have grown up in different cultures or socio-economic strata, or come from different racial, religious, or educational backgrounds. Research suggests that regardless of sexual preference, most people today struggle to reconcile a longing for intimacy with a desire for independence, to attain a dynamic balance between attachment and autonomy (Peplau, 1981; Willi, 1982). Still, lesbians and gay men in relationships face additional challenges unique to them. Simply being two people of the same sex who live as a minority in a heterosexual society has special interactional implications for the couple, especially in the area of attempting to achieve a balance between closeness and separateness. Without fully appreciating the special psychosocial situation such couples face as they strive to develop coping mechanisms for dealing with the unique aspects of their lives together, the assessment and treatment of gay couples cannot adequately be carried out.

Some innovative theoretical work taking into account the effects of environmental pressures on personality formation and couple interaction among lesbians and gay men has gradually begun to appear. Gonsiorek (1982) has noted the ways in which homosexuals with diverse personality structures may develop similar "characterological-appearing overlays" due to the similar kinds of stressful situations to which they have to adapt. Krestan and Bepko (1980), operating from a comprehensive family systems model, have described how forces acting upon lesbian couples by the larger society, as well as from the lesbian community, create interactional, that is, fusion-separation problems in couples. A group of clinicians and researchers based in California (Lindenbaum et al., 1982) have been developing a conceptual framework combining an object relations and family systems approach for identifying the salient clinical and theoretical issues in working with lesbians and their social/familial contexts. The systems perspective seems to be particularly relevant in formulating productive interventions for same-sex couples because, as Krestan and Bepko explain (p. 277), it depends upon an "awareness of the problem inherent in the couple's attempt to define the rules of their relationship within the context of a larger system in which no rules relating to them exist."

THE PROBLEM OF BOUNDARIES

Minuchin (1974) and other prominent family therapists refer to the "rules" defining who participates in the relationship and how they do so as the "boundaries" of the subsystem. The problem of defining the inner and outer boundaries of the dyad includes such questions as how close to each other can the partners become before they will lose their individuality, and to what extent a couple should separate itself from the larger system outside. Each couple must find an appropriate position on a continuum between total fusion and rigid separation.

If dyadic fusion occurs, the partners form a symbiotic unit, closing themselves off tightly from outsiders. In a sense, this is exactly what is expected to happen in the "falling in love" and "honeymoon period" of most relationships. However, if this situation continues, it may lead to a loss of ego boundaries, dissolution of the self, and suppression of all aggressive, and often, sexual drives.

At the other extreme are those couples who, through anxiety about loss of the self and fear of intimacy, maintain rigid separation between each other. Meanwhile, extradyadically, the boundaries are often diffused. Relatives, friends, children, sexual intimacy with a third person or a symptom such as alcoholism is triangled into the relationship to limit the extent of close contact with the partner. Couples who have difficulties in setting boundaries typically present patterns of cycles of fusion and unrelatedness, alternating reactive separation, continual open conflict, or psychosomatic impairment of one partner.

If, taking this model, the same-sex couple is viewed as a subsystem functioning within the context of a larger system composed of co-workers, family of origin, and friends, it becomes clear that a model of satisfying relatedness involves the formation both by the couple and by the larger system of boundaries that are clear, respected, and flexible. Within the dyad the partners retain their unique identities while, at the same time, the outer boundaries are well delineated. The partners have a life of their own and establish clear lines between themselves and parents and children, between themselves and extra-dyadic friends and/or lovers. It also becomes clear, as Krestan and Bepko point out, that the primary difficulty the committed same-sex dyad faces in striving to define the "rules" relative to their relationship is that the boundaries go largely unrecognized by the larger system. Thus, the tendency toward fusion or reactive separation in same-sex couples results in part from attempts by the couple to maintain a subsystem within a larger system which typically treats their relationship as if it were invisible or pathological.

SAME-SEX COUPLES IN THE HETEROSEXUAL SYSTEM

In our society, the traditional marriage is the only socially supported model for establishing and maintaining long-term sexual and affectional relationships. The heterosexual relationship is usually cemented by legal and religious sanctions, validated by a formal engagement and a public marriage ceremony, and upon event of dissolution, requires a formal divorce process. The legal commitment of matrimony usually means that the couple will take up a joint residence, share property in common, follow socially prescribed roles as husband and wife, bear and raise children, and so forth. Since this heterosexual model has been developed largely on the basis of gender role expectations, it is not particularly functional for partners of the same gender. Homosexual couples have to define their roles in the relative absence of models of same-sex intimacy. Raised by heterosexual parents, lacking marriage manuals and images of conjugal bliss on film or T.V., faced with a situation where gay couples who do develop successful relationships are seldom visible (Toder, 1978), unable to acquire the socially sanctioned same-sex dating experiences equivalent to that which non-gay men and women get with each other during adolescence (Moses & Hawkins, Jr., 1982), and lacking structured courtship rituals (Antony, 1982), gay couples, as one author puts it (Berzon, 1979), have had to "wing it" when it comes to creating workable love and life relationships.

For many same-sex couples, being committed means sharing a living space while, for others, separate housing is preferred. To some couples, commitment may mean pooling resources; for others not. Some couples expect monogamy; others prefer allowing for sex with other partners. Some couples enact gender-typed roles; some do not (Bell & Weinberg, 1978; Jay & Young, 1979; Peplau & Gordon, 1982; Saghir & Robins, 1975; Tanner, 1978). There have been an increasing number of studies trying to identify what patterns exist in gay relationships (Harry, in press; Larson, 1982; Peplau, Padesky, & Hamilton, 1982). For example, Peplau and her associates have found that the balance of power in lesbian relationships affects the degree to which individuals are satisfied with them; women in more equal power relationships report greater satisfaction. Silverstein (1982) recently identified two general categories of gay men—excitement seekers and home-builders—with most gay men being a combination of both, but each man usually motivated more in one direction than the other. Longlasting relationships, he says, are generally of the home-builder type, and domestic-type lovers often live the same life-style as do heterosexual couples in the community. McWhirter and Mattison (1983) found that homosexual male couples living together go through stages of development from a romantic, idealized "enthrallment" in the beginning to a settled, comfortable, more mature enthrallment after about twenty years together.

While these studies suggesting possible patterns in lesbian and gay male relationships are interesting, what may be most important for the purposes of this article is that without the gender-role structure of the traditional heterosexual model, the form of dyadic interactions becomes an important variable in working with same-sex couples. While many couples experience the lack of clear-cut gender-role expectations as liberating, it can also be a source of confusion. Once the heterosexual model is ostensibly discarded, much energy can be spent on difficulties arising from differing interpretations by the partners of what constitutes an appropriate and desirable interaction in a committed love relationship. Because so many areas of the relationship are uncharted by traditional expectations, there may be a greater tendency to put myths of romantic love and fantasies about how the relationship should be conducted into unspoken "contracts" which need to be translated if the couple is to form a workable relationship.

LACK OF EXTERNAL SUPPORTS

The couple struggles with this challenge to create satisfying intradyadic arrangements without the social supports usually enjoyed by the heterosexual couple. In same-sex relationships, the absence of legal ceremony means that individuals may move rapidly into commitment and be considered by themselves and others in the gay community as a couple. They do so without any kind of legal protection, religious mandate, or public validation concerning their behavior so that their relationship is much more vulnerable than that of a non-gay couple. It can be dissolved without filing for divorce. If one of the partners in a committed same-sex relationship should die, the remaining partner is often isolated because of the failure of society to recognize the validity of the relationship. Because they are not legally family, they may not be allowed into an intensive care setting. After the partner's death, they may be kept from retaining any of the partner's possessions, from attending the funeral, and may be prevented from being a beneficiary even though the partner so specified in the will (Curry & Clifford, 1980).

There are other less dramatic but equally real examples of how difficult it may be for same-sex couples to form firm extradyadic boundaries when supports available to other couples in society are not available to them. Because there are few socially acceptable mechanisms for mourning the ending of a relationship that was looked upon by society as non-existent or an expression of deviant behavior, a gay person may move from one relationship into another having less completely separated from the prior partner. Same-sex relationships may also be more vulnerable to post-honeymoon crises because the absence of any sanctifying ritual—including an actual "honeymoon"—means that the necessity for establishing the relationship as both special and binding lies almost completely with the couple. When the diminution in intensity and sense of exclusive oneness that generally occurs in all relationships is experienced by the same-sex couple, it may be taken as a sign by one partner or both that something is severely wrong with the relationship. One woman who had previously been in a heterosexual marriage said that since she had to make so many social sacrifices to be in a lesbian relationship, she felt that it had to be perfect. Two men, both of whom had formerly been in heterosexual marriages, noticed that the same kinds of little problems that they used to tolerate with their wives, now in a gay relationship, seemed to take on much greater meaning because the relationship seemed so much less socially protected.

These pressures are exacerbated by the fact that same-sex couples live in a climate of anti-homosexuality. Not only do they work to sustain their relationships without the given "rules" and positive sanctions available to heterosexual couples. They do so in a society which manifests the deep dread and emphatic disapproval of same-sex eroticism and intimacy referred to as homophobia. As

Goffman noted in his early studies on stigma (1963), homosexuality is seen as symptomatic of a moral failing. Furthermore, the socialization of the homosexual, as Maylon points out (1982, p. 60), "nearly always involves an internalization of the mythology and opprobrium which characterizes current attitudes toward homosexuality." The anti-gay jokes to which all children are exposed in their formative years are but one example of this process.

This situation is complicated by the fact that, as Goffman points out, the moral stigma of homosexuality differs from other physical and racial types of stigma in its degree of visibility. While the visibly stigmatized are "discredited"—most of those with physical handicaps, or belonging to a minority racial group cannot hide their stigma—those considered to have a moral failing, whom Goffman calls "discreditable," can hide their stigma by "passing" as "normal" among other normals. "Coming out," that is, acknowledging oneself as homosexual, and from there, letting various others know, is a difficult process which never ends as long as one is living in a heterosexual world where the assumption is always that one is "straight."

THE EFFECTS OF HOMOPHOBIA AND THE COMING OUT PROCESS ON SAME-SEX COUPLES

The stress that results when one or both members of a couple are open about their sexual preference is another area unique to same-sex relationships. Not only do the intrapsychic consequences of adapting to a stigmatized identity tend to bring more anxiety, fear, and friction into the relationship, but also the couple often experiences pressure to maintain secrecy about their relationship—never to be seen at public functions together or to show any natural affection for one another in places where, otherwise, it would seem entirely appropriate. If partners are at different stages or in different situations in "coming out," the decisions that each makes in negotiating relationships with the larger system will directly affect the other. It often may constitute additional pressure towards fusion or reactive separation.

Taking a position about one's homosexuality usually triggers a chain reaction of responses that may impede or support the couple's strivings to maintain boundaries. Many jobs and professional affiliations require some amount of socializing where one is expected to bring a spouse or date. Whether a gay person chooses not to go to such a function, to go alone, or to take her/his partner and risk revealing their sexual preference, will have an effect on both the couple interaction and the relationships with peers. The same is true with regard to talking about one's partner with co-workers. To come out in this manner has been compared to the "demand bid" in bridge (Krestan & Bepko, 1981, pp. 250-251) whereby the people told feel compelled to make some kind of re-active response that goes beyond the level of intimacy the gay person may have wanted. To the extent that the couple feels they must cut off meaningful professional and social connections, they are more likely to feel the pressure of it's "the two of us against the world" phenomenon. If one member of the couple would like to attend professional functions and the other doesn't feel comfort-able doing so, or if one partner wants to give a party for co-work-ers at home and expects the other to pretend that he or she doesn't live there or is "just a roommate," confusion, anger, and depres-sion are almost bound to appear.

In one lesbian couple who consulted me with regard to anxiety and depression, one woman, Judy—both were lawyers working in different firms—wanted to go to office parties together while the other woman, Pat, did not. It turned out that Judy felt Pat was ashamed of her. It also became clear over time that Pat, who claimed initially that after two previous relationships with women, both lasting over six years, she didn't think of herself as a lesbian because "I just happen to be with a woman now," was living with a great deal of internalized homophobia and didn't really believe the relationship was viable because she was sure her parents, to whom she was not open, could never accept it.

Same-sex couples usually experience the most intense difficul-ties when coming out to the family of origin of one member. In contrast with families of other minority members, they have not shared their stigmatized identity. Whether they're told directly or not, they may react with a mixture of denial, horror, guilt, and/or the kind of acceptance that allows everyone to believe that a per-son in a same-sex relationship never really leaves the family at all. Holidays often present good examples of the tendency for bound-aries to be ignored or violated in the face of family pressure.

One couple, John and Robert, who entered therapy because they were continually "fighting over nothing," only recently were able to spend their first major holiday together after six years of spending holidays with Robert's parents supposedly because his parents accepted them and John's did not. However, on these visits, Robert's parents would continue to ask Robert in subtle ways about whether he wouldn't like to date and would treat John as if he, at the age of 36, was a temporary friend who would be their ally in helping Robert to "settle down" and raise a family. When they finally decided to give their relationship priority and to begin creating their own family traditions, Robert's mother finally burst out, "Your being gay is the biggest disappointment in your father's and my life," and took a much more hostile position. In this case, both men, by virtue of clarifying the boundaries around their relationship, must deal at least temporarily with being cut off from their families of origin more than they would like to be.

To the extent that same-sex couples have difficulties in developing satisfying spheres of integration with families of origin, with co-workers, and with friends, they may feel additional cause to expect the relationship to make up for the sense of isolation and alienation they experience. Because of the extra sense of social vulnerability, couples may not want to look at areas of difference for fear that it means things aren't working.

Rather than using anger in the service of emotional separation, couples may be indirectly hostile or avoid anger at all lest it signal the end. Because of the lack of tangible legal, socially sanctioned bonds, the threat of independence—spending time in outside interests or the desire for increased privacy—may be heightened. Insecurities stemming from these situations should not be taken by the therapist as an indicator of overdependence without considering the stresses consequent to the unique pressures on same-sex couples. Couples must be helped to understand the vicious circles implicit in their situations. The more enmeshed and turned in on themselves the couple becomes, the greater they will feel the need to escape the intensity of the relationship. Because the same-sex couple often must spend greater amounts of energy defining boundaries in order to maintain their relationship and private couple space and, because for the same-sex couple differentiation is not countered by external forces supporting the survival of the partnership, any energy spent on more individuated behavior may be seen as tipping the scales toward dissolution. There may be a tendency to resolve conflicts around merging and differentiation by reactive separation, by ending the relationship, often prematurely, or by triangling a third person in as a way of saying "I'm separate from you," as though the only way not to be totally defined by the partner is either to split up or take another lover.

DIFFERENCES BETWEEN LESBIAN AND GAY MALE RELATIONSHIPS

It has been suggested that lesbian and gay male couples respond to these systemic pressures in different ways which reflect differences in the socialization of women and men (Krestan & Bepko, 1981). Women, whether heterosexual or homosexual, are rewarded early for clinging and the development of relationship skills whereby they learn to merge their own identities with others by making the needs and feelings of others their own (Chodorow, 1978), and to equate sex with love so that they feel they must be in love in order to legitimize their sexual activity. Men, on the other hand, whether heterosexual or homosexual, are conditioned by society to make relationship skills secondary to the ability to be differentiated, to win, achieve, earn, make sexual conquests not necessarily associated with being in love, and to exhibit strength and self-control by not showing emotion (McClandish, 1982). One study comparing heterosexual and homosexual men and women on the importance they give to different characteristics of relationships (Peplau, 1981) found differences based on sex to be more significant than those based on sexual preference, with women expressing more need for openness, sharing, and communication than men. In his work on heterosexual couples, Willi (1982) has observed that a man who will speak openly about his weaknesses in individual sessions will hold himself back and assume a much more controlled, balanced pose in couple therapy. Conversely, the woman partner, who in the single therapy sessions demonstrated a constructive approach to a working relationship, behaved much more regressively and passively in the common therapy session. Work with heterosexual couples suggests that women have a tendency to live below their potential and to relinquish their self-realization in a couple relationship whereas men, although looking more independent and distant in the relationship, often tend to be more devastated and unable to take care of themselves if the relationship ends.

It follows, then, that faced with conflicts around merging and differentiation which are intensified by the adaptational task of being homosexual in a heterosexual world, lesbian couples with very little practice at self-definition and autonomy in relationships, may tend towards fusion. Gay male couples, on the other hand, who have less practice in nurturing skills and who have often been discouraged from appearing weak or dependent, may tend more towards reactive distance. Two women who have broken up and gotten back together several times emphasize again and again how much more autonomous they are able to be when they're apart. Only gradually are they beginning to believe that they can both develop their own individuality while remaining in the relationship. Two men who were both previously in heterosexual relationships, find themselves competing over everything from sexual prowess and earning power to who is the better father. They are only beginning to allow each other to see their vulnerabilities, to ask for and to give nurturing and affection.

Even with these examples, however, I believe it would be ill advised to do too much generalizing about the differences between lesbian and gay male relationships when we still have so little solid research on same-sex couples. What seems most clear at this stage of investigation is that both gay men and lesbians in couples experience intensified social pressures which complicate their attempts to achieve a workable balance between oneness and differentiation, between attachment and autonomy, between sharing and individuation.

CLINICAL ISSUES AND POLICY IMPLICATIONS

The worker's attitude toward same-sex couple's difficulties in achieving this balance will greatly affect the success of the therapy or counseling. Too often clinicians automatically assume that problems around forming boundaries in same-sex couples indicate intrapsychic pathology resulting from homosexuality *per se* rather than taking into account how these difficulties may be related to normal adaptational mechanisms of all same-sex relationships. This does not mean that the clinician should necessarily engage in "blaming society" therapy or encourage politicizing of the issue of sexual preference when it is being used to avoid dealing with issues of intimacy and separation/individuation or the pain engendered by nonrecognition or total rejection by family, co-workers, or friends. Same-sex couples need to be helped to distinguish between exogogenous and internalized homophobia and to see all the ways in which they may maintain a victim attitude or provoke and perpetuate their social isolation. However, in order to facilitate this process, the therapist must be fully aware and appreciative of the unique psychosocial pressures that same-sex couples face, while helping them to reframe the relationship as one that is inherently worthy of being valued and capable of being maintained, and not one that is inherently sick and unworkable. Many couples will be relieved to discover that the difficulties they are experiencing are common to other couples and will be responsive to looking at how issues of merging and differentiation get played out in their particular relationship. The formation of a same-sex couples' group can be especially helpful as a place for couples to explore solutions to common problems: the coming out process, the rules of participation in the relationship, and the efforts to form clear boundaries around the relationship while maintaining individuality within it.

Clinicians who work with same-sex couples need to have a thorough knowledge of psychodynamic and family system principles, a sophisticated understanding of atypical socialization and stigmatization with particular reference to identity problems related to homophobia and coming out, a familiarity with the lesbian and gay male subcultures, and a belief that homosexual relationships are valid and viable. In the last case, there seems little to suggest any change in attitude or policy since 1979 when Masters and Johnson noted that if the homosexual population expected the worst from health-care professionals, they would rarely be disappointed (p. 247). DeCrescenza and McGill's study (1978) of the attitude of mental health professionals toward homosexuality found homophobia to be the most prevalent among social workers with 43% of the respondents saying they believed gays and lesbians should be tolerated only if they don't publicly show their way of life. Since living as a couple is probably the most public way that a homosexual can show his or her way of life, it is difficult to see how same-sex couples can hope for adequate help from most social work professionals. Although being a homosexual does not guarantee freedom from homophobic or heterosexist bias, it does seem, as has been suggested (Potter & Darty, 1981), that lesbian and gay male couples who seek help would be better served by social service agencies that do not automatically bar acknowledged homosexuals from their professional staff. Such a situation not only contributes to creating an oppressive atmosphere for gay clients, but it also deprives agencies of people who could serve as an important resource for other staff members (Woodman & Lenna, 1980). In any case, greater attention to these issues via research, policy, supervision and training seminars may prove beneficial not only to those gay men and women who seek greater integrity and growth in their partnerships, but to the integrity and growth of the mental health professions, as well.

CONCLUSIONS

This article expresses the position that systemic pressures which cause the boundaries around the same-sex couple to be ignored or trespassed must be taken into consideration if the full range of developmental conditions which lead to symptomatic adaptations in lesbian and gay male relationships are to be understood and adequately treated. While recognizing that homosexuals may exhibit the same diversity of character types and personality disorders as heterosexuals, this approach focuses on the interactional consequences of biased socialization. It regards the stigmatization that accompanies homosexuality and the pressures that attend the coming out process to be salient variables in the development of dysfunctional relationships among gay men and lesbians. Finally, I have taken the position that the clinician working with same-sex couples needs to be fully cognizant of their unique difficulties in creating respected boundaries. Only by understanding and dealing with these difficulties can the members of the couple achieve a more satisfying relationship with each other and with the heterosexual world in which they live.

REFERENCES

Bell, A. & Weinberg, M. *Homosexualities: A study of diversity among men and women.* New York: Simon & Schuster, 1978.

Berzon, B. Achieving success as a gay couple. In B. Berzon & R. Leighton (Eds.), *Positively gay: New approaches in gay life.* Millibrae, CA: Celestial Arts, 1978.

Chodorow, N. *The reproduction of mothering: Psychoanalysis and the sociology of gender.* Berkeley & Los Angeles: University of California Press, 1978.

Curry, H. & Clifford, D. *A legal guide for lesbian and gay couples.* Nolo Press Book, 1980.

DeCrescenza, T. & McGill, C. *Homophobia: A study of the attitudes of mental health professionals toward homosexuality.* Unpublished master's thesis. University of Southern California, School of Social Work, 1978.

Dulaney, D. & Kelly, J. Improving services to gay and lesbian clients, *Social Work*, 1982, 27(2), 178-183.

Goffman, E. *Stigma: Notes on a spoiled identity*. Englewood Cliffs, N.J.: Prentice-Hall, 1963.

Gonsiorek, J. The use of diagnostic concepts in working with gay and lesbian populations. In J. Gonsiorek (Ed.), *Homosexuality and psychotherapy: A practitioner's handbook of affirmative models*. New York: Haworth Press, 1982.

Harry, J. Gay male and lesbian family relationships. In E. Macklin (Ed.), *Contemporary families and alternative lifestyles: Handbook on research and theory*. Beverly Hills, CA: Sage, in press.

Jay, K. & Young, A. *The gay report*. New York: Summit Books, 1979.

Krestan, J. & Bepko, C. The problem of fusion in the lesbian relationship. *Family Process*, 1980, 19, 277-289.

Larson, P. Gay male relationships. In W. Paul, J. Weinrich, J. Gonsiorek, & Mary Hotvedt (Eds.), *Homosexuality: Social, Psychological, and Biological Issues*. Beverly Hills, CA.: Sage Publications, 1982.

Lindenbaum, J., Blum, A., DeMonteflores, C., Feinstein, N., Lyons, T. & Weston, A. Lesbian relationships in their social, familial, and clinical contexts. Course presented at 59th annual meeting of the American Orthopsychiatric Association, San Francisco, April 3, 1982.

Marmor, J. Overview: The multiple roots of homosexual behavior. In J. Marmor (Ed.), *Homosexual behavior: A modern reappraisal*. New York: Basic Books, Inc., 1980.

Masters, W. & Johnson, V. *Homosexuality in perspective*. Boston: Little Brown, 1979.

Maylon, A. Psychotherapeutic implications of internalized homophobia in gay men. In J. Gonsiorek (Ed.), *Homosexuality and psychotherapy: A practitioner's handbook of affirmative models*. New York: Haworth Press, 1982.

McClandish, B. Therapeutic issues with lesbian couples. In J. Gonsiorek (Ed.), *Homosexuality and psychotherapy: A practitioner's handbook of affirmative models*. New York: Haworth Press, 1982.

McWhirter, D. & Mattison, A. *Stages: A developmental study of homosexual male couples*. New York: St. Marten's, in press.

Minuchin, S. *Families and family therapy*. Cambridge: Harvard University Press, 1974.

Moses, A. & Hawkins, Jr., R. Lesbians' and gay mens' relationships, In *Counseling lesbian and gay men: A life-issues approach*. St. Louis: The C.V. Mosby Co., 1982.

Peplau, L. What homosexuals want in relationships. *Psychology Today*, 1981, 15(3), 28-38.

Peplau, L., Cochran, S., Rook, K., & Padesky, C. Loving women: Attachment and autonomy in lesbian relationships. *Journal of Social Issues*, 1978, 34(3), 7-27.

Peplau, L. & Gordon, S. The intimate relationships of lesbian and gay men. In E. R. Allgeier & N. B. McCormick (Eds.), *Gender roles and sexual behavior*. Palo Alto, CA: Mayfield, 1982.

Peplau, L., Padesky, C. & Hamilton, M. Satisfaction in lesbian relationships. In L. Peplau & R. Jones (Eds.), *Symposium on homosexual couples, Special issue of Journal of Homosexuality*, Winter, 1982, 7(2), 23-37.

Potter, S. & Darty, T. Social work and the invisible minority: An exploration of lesbianism. *Social Work*, 1981, 26(3), 187-192.

Saghir, M. & Robins, E. *Male and female homosexuality: A comprehensive investigation*. Baltimore: Williams & Witkins, 1973.

Silverstein, C. *Man to man: Gay couples in America*. New York: Quill, 1982.

Tanner, D. *The lesbian couple*. Lexington, Mass.: D.C. Heath, 1978.

Toder, N. Couples: The hidden segment of the gay world. *Journal of Homosexuality*, 1978, 3, 331-343.

Willi, J. *Couples in collusion*. New York: Jason Aronson, 1982.

Woodman, N. & Lenna, H. *Counseling with gay men and women: A guide for facilitating positive lifestyles*. San Francisco: Jossey-Bass, 1980.

The Sage Model for Serving
Older Lesbians and Gay Men

Morgan Gwenwald

There are over 35,600,000 people who are 60 years old or older in the United States.[1] Kinsey's estimate of incidence of homosexuality in the general population applied to this figure suggests that there may be 3,560,000 older gay men and lesbians in the U.S. This figure is greater than the total number of people living in nursing homes in this country.

Senior Action in a Gay Environment (SAGE) is one model of a community's efforts to recognize this population and provide services to it. This paper examines the history of SAGE and its efforts to serve this community of older gay men and lesbians.

The last ten years have been a period of intensive growth in the area of gerontology. We have also seen, since the mid 60s, a demand for unbiased examination of issues concerning gay men and lesbians.

These developments have resulted in a trickle of information, appearing in journals, about elderly gay men and lesbians.[2] Most of these articles have presented little more than exploratory research, posing questions and problems. They have also focused almost exclusively on gay males, which is common, historically, throughout the literature on homosexuality. Only in the past few years have some efforts been made to do more extensive research in the area of gay and lesbian aging.[3] A major research effort on older lesbians has just been completed by Chris Almvig. That, along with Raymond M. Berger's work, represents the most comprehensive research on the subject thus far.[4]

Although it is far from definitive, the information currently available on elderly gay men and lesbians challenges the prevailing perceptions of this population. Prevailing stereotypes of the older gay male—that he has an unsatisfactory sex life, that he associates increasingly with heterosexuals—have been challenged by Kelly's study of 241 gay men in Los Angeles.[5] What does emerge from the literature is a description of individuals who are self-sufficient, have a positive self-image and have developed a wide range of skills for survival.

The people who come to SAGE in most part confirm this positive image. Our sense is that, for a variety of reasons, they may be better equipped to cope with the societal aspects of the aging process. They have most likely already dealt with societal rejection and oppression stemming from their sexuality. Kimmel found a "conscious preparation for self-reliance during the later years, experience in all of the relevant skills for maintaining oneself and one's home."[6]

We believe this to be especially true for lesbians as compared to heterosexual women. Unlike many heterosexual women who have lived their lives within traditional roles, many lesbians have developed a wide range of skills necessary for daily living. Whereas heterosexual men and women engaged in traditional roles develop only half of the skills needed for survival, gay men and lesbians usually have to learn the whole range of skills necessary for living (e.g., balancing a budget, arranging transportation, preparing food, and earning a living). At the point that a heterosexual person may lose a mate, he or she is faced with a whole range of difficulties related to daily living skills, in addition to the problems of bereavement.

Both the helping professions and the gay community itself have begun to recognize the special strengths and the special needs of aging lesbians and gay men.

HISTORY

In 1977 a small group of gay men and lesbians in New York City, noting the relative absence of older gay men and lesbians in the community's groups and activities, began to meet in an effort to examine the issues of gay aging. Some of the founding members were older, or friends of older lesbians and gay men, and knew first-hand the kinds of isolation and problems with which this population had to struggle. One of the early goals of this group, and still a powerful vision for many people working with SAGE, was a home for senior gay men and lesbians. They turned their efforts first, though, to more manageable tasks and the organization of the group. By 1979 SAGE became incorporated as a tax-exempt non-profit organization.

Some of the founders of SAGE had experienced working with aging in gerontological and other social service programs. Their influence guided SAGE, from its inception, toward the development of an organization that would operate and provide services in a professional manner. A pilot program was developed, and three grant proposals were written in 1979. With this, the stage was set for rapid growth of programming and outreach into the gay and aging community.

SAGE was quite successful in its initial fundraising efforts in the foundation arena. In 1980 it became the first gay organization in the northeast to secure a grant from the United Way.[7] Other grants awarded, and now almost depleted, came from Community Board #2 Federal Archives Fund and the New York Community Trust.[8] Because of its successful fundraising in both the private and public sector, SAGE has been able to hire three staff people. SAGE currently has a full-time Executive Director, full-time Administrative Assistant, and a 4/5 time Coordinator of Direct Services (MSW social workers).

In the absence of a mandate from a governmental agency or an established religious group, SAGE realizes it is unwise to depend on foundation and public support. Liberal foundations, interested in pilot programs, often are less willing or able to provide funds for ongoing operating expenses.

Now SAGE is turning more toward the gay community itself for support—through direct mail campaigns, cocktail parties, and other fundraising events. What may be potential limits of this strategy are suggested by the San Francisco Gay Care Study on fundraising efforts of Bay Area gay groups.[9] Its finding show that gay organizations need to understand the size of their community base and strive not to deplete the resources of that community. Where more and more organizations make demands for economic support from essentially the same people, a certain amount of tensions and problems begin to occur.

The principle way of seeking support from the gay community without depleting its economic resources is through the use of volunteers. Rather than raising funds for hiring additional staff, or paying for certain services, volunteers can supplement core staff and often provide professional services free of charge (e.g., assistance with bookkeeping, legal advice). This strategy has been especially successful at SAGE, which has a large membership of retired persons, with a rich background of skills to share.

This structure—a small number of paid staff working with a large body of volunteer staff—has become the standard mode of operation for most gay service organizations nationwide, including gay counseling centers, gay V.D. clinics, and gay community centers. As such, it is worth examining in some detail how this kind of organization functions.

STRUCTURE

The activities of SAGE are governed by a Board of Directors, made up of 24 individuals, elected for three year terms. As SAGE has grown, so too has the scope of activities which the Board is asked to address. Initially this board was composed mainly of volunteers from the various committees. At this point, the composition of the Board is shifting to include a number of experts and professionals from the gay community in order to provide greater expertise and leadership in areas of funding, expansion and goal-setting. Increasingly, older lesbians and gay men are themselves Board members.

SAGE's Executive Director works with the Executive Committee and the Board of Directors. The main function of the executive director is overall development and coordination of SAGE, especially in areas of funding.

The Coordinator of Direct Services, the other paid professional position at SAGE, is responsible to the Executive Director and the Board. The main functions of this person are to develop outreach programs, coordinate educational activities, and provide support and direction to the volunteers.

Volunteers learn about SAGE from a variety of sources including gay organizations, aging organizations, outreach at events, media exposure and through word-of-mouth. Many of these people have no previous volunteer experience. They come to SAGE because the specific issues of aging touch their own concerns, or the experiences of friends and/or family. The myth that gay men are unable and unwilling to cope with the aging process is challenged by the work of SAGE, since more than half of all SAGE volunteers are men, and range in age from their 20s through 80s.

Volunteers work in one or more of the seven committees that provide structure for SAGE's volunteer force. Two persons—one woman and one man, whenever possible—chair each committee. Their leadership is considered crucial to SAGE's success. All the committee co-chairs meet regularly together with the staff.

The Assessor's Committee is composed of social workers and other helping professionals. They do intake assessments of the older people who have requested friendly visiting or other direct service assistance from SAGE. If it is determined that a friendly visitor should be assigned they make the referral and then provide case management and back-up support for the friendly visitor. Where appropriate they make referrals to agencies and organizations. SAGE does not attempt to duplicate services but strives to fill in the gaps in services provided by traditional agencies.

Friendly Visitors make a commitment to visit, on a regular basis, with an older lesbian or gay man who may be homebound, or needs assistance with activities such as shopping or trips to the doctor. These volunteers receive training on issues of aging, social service and gay resources. Like the Assessor's Committee, the Friendly Visitors meet monthly for peer supervision and assignment of new cases.

There is also a Telephone Reassurance Service provided by the Friendly Visitors Committee. This is one area of direct services that older members of SAGE can participate in who perhaps cannot take on the responsibility of a weekly visiting schedule.

These two committees, the Assessors and the Friendly Visitors are the heart of the services that SAGE provides to older lesbians and gay men. Through the combined efforts and skills of these two groups, SAGE is able to provide weekly support to a large number of people.

Elliot is one example of an elderly man who came to rely on these services. He was suffering from a progressively debilitating disease and confined in a medical facility for several months. When it was obvious he would never be leaving, his former lover and only link to the outside world planned to leave town. Before leaving, the man contacted SAGE about Elliot and a Friendly Visitor was assigned. The Friendly Visitor traveled to a remote part of the city every week for two years to see Elliot and visit for an hour or more. The volunteer from SAGE became the only person outside of hospital staff that Elliot ever saw, the only friend and contact with the world and his past. Due to the volunteer's constant presence, Elliot's needs were likely better attended to than if he was alone in the institution. More important, though, was Elliot's contact with someone who was there for him and cared about him.

Jill is another who has derived help from these services. She was an isolated elderly woman who called for SAGE for Friendly Visiting Service. After an assessment period, it was determined that she didn't really require a Friendly Visitor, but phone reassurance was extended to her. After a few months of regular phone contact and encouragement, Jill attended one of SAGE's monthly socials, knowing that the phone contact would be present. She attended a second social and then started traveling all the way from Brooklyn to Greenwich Village to attend the weekly women's 50-plus rap group. Through the support of SAGE staff and opportunities for socialization, she has decreased her own isolation and found new friends. Her self-respect and confidence have improved as has the quality of her life away from SAGE as well.

OTHER COMMITTEES

The Group Services Committee organizes and carries out a monthly social event. A social typically includes a sit-down dinner and live music and dancing, organized around a theme. Other activities have included a boat tour of Manhattan and an outdoor picnic. At a recent social we celebrated the 50th anniversary of two of our members. Many new volunteers choose to work here in order to get a feel for the organization. Group Services is also well suited for people who cannot commit a regular or large amount of time to SAGE but can show up and help at a particular event. The socials reach a large population of older lesbians and gay men who are self-sufficient but may not have many options for socializing. Should they encounter situations in their lives that require other levels of support, they are already connected to SAGE.

The Communications Committee handles much of SAGE's publicity and outreach. The Committee produces and publishes four newsletters a year for a mailing list of over 3,500, a monthly calendar of events, fliers and press releases for SAGE activities. Most of the Communication Committee volunteers have experience in publicity, writing, editing, typesetting or computer programming. SAGE's Speakers Bureau is also coordinated by the Communications Committee. It has the involvement of many of the older members of SAGE and provides speakers for gay groups and aging groups wanting to know more about SAGE and the experiences of older lesbians and gay men. Some members of the Speakers Bureau are also available to conduct in-service training sessions for agencies that want to learn more about gay men and lesbians and the issues of aging in that community.

The Workshop Committee runs a writer's group (which produced a book, *SAGE Writings*), separate "rap" groups for men and women, a drama workshop, a film discussion group, a nutrition group and a travel group. As new needs and interests arise, SAGE tries to develop new groups to meet those needs. A monthly square dance, ball room dancing lessons, a sing-along group and bowling group are currently in the planning stages.

The final two committees provide organizational support to SAGE: Financial Planning and Intake and Matching. Financial Planning assists in directing SAGE's funding efforts and expenditures. The Intake and Matching Committee coordinates the flow of new volunteers into SAGE. Each month members of this committee interview prospective volunteers, offer them a formal orientation to the organization, and refer them to specific committees.

Volunteers also help with an enormous amount of the day-to-day office work. Their assistance is crucial for large bulk mailings and in keeping up with the ever growing mailing lists. Many people, who are retired or employed part-time, volunteer part of their day time hours to help out in the office.

In its four years of operation, SAGE has provided service for over 400 gay men and lesbian elders in New York City. It has served as a model for other groups in the U.S. in such cities as Washington, D.C., Los Angeles, Denver and Philadelphia.

A major concern for these groups is locating the population they're committed to serve. After all, elderly gays and lesbians have been under more cultural pressure to internalize society's negative attitudes towards homosexuality than their younger counterparts have, and may be more hesitant to identify themselves as homosexual when in a vulnerable state, for example, when faced with debilitating illnesses.

Accordingly, SAGE serves two fairly distinct populations. One is the larger group of ambulatory, self-sufficient older lesbians and gay men who look to SAGE for social, educational and similar services. Many of this group also serve as volunteers in various capacities in the organization as well.

The other group is seemingly smaller, and far more difficult to locate—the isolated homebound population. This group is by definition very isolated, both physically and sometimes emotionally. They are in most instances cut off from the sources of information normally available through the lesbian and gay community, newspapers, bar notices, bookstores, etc. Their access to other sources of information (bulletin boards in senior centers for instance) is often equally limited. There may not be anyone near them that they share their sexual orientation with. Our experience has been that in most cases this elderly population has maintained a fairly high level of secrecy regarding their sexuality, throughout their lives. Very often their support networks are relatively small, discrete circles of friends and lovers. As they age and this network shrinks due to people moving away and dying, if they become homebound, they are very likely to become isolated as well.

Often they are quite reticent to discuss their feelings with a social worker. In at least one case, a social worker at a non-gay geriatric center spent years gaining the trust of the client before she, the client, felt comfortable discussing her sexual orientation.

SAGE is currently developing a Pilot Outreach Plan to be concentrated in Greenwich Village, New York City. Two of the main focuses of outreach efforts will be through the straight media (local papers, radio shows, cable TV, public service announcements, etc) and through service providers. Besides contacting all hospitals, nursing homes, meals-on-wheels type programs, and social service agencies, SAGE will be offering training to providers in issues affecting older lesbians and gay men. It is hoped that these providers may become sources of information for their clients.

For those working with elderly lesbians and gay men, developing new and creative ways to reach out to this population is perhaps the most worthwhile and challenging task for the future.

NOTES

1. United States Bureau of the Census, U.S. Department of Commerce, 1980.

2. Douglas C. Kimmel, "Adult Development and Aging: A Gay Perspective," *Journal of Social Issues*, Vol 34, #3, 1978, pp. 113-131. Del Martin and Phyllis Lyon, "The Older Lesbian," *Positively Gay*, Betty Berzon ed., Celestial Arts, 1979, pp. 134-145. Martin S. Weinberg & Colin J. Williams, "Age," *Male Homosexuals*, Penguin Books, 1975, pp. 309-317.

3. Raymond M. Berger, "Psychological Adaptation of the Older Homosexual Male," *Journal of Homosexuality*, Vol 5 (3), Spring 1980, pp. 161-175. Douglas C. Kimmel, "Ad-

justments to Aging Among Gay Men," *Positively Gay,* Betty Berzon, ed., Celestial Arts, 1979. Fred A. Minnigerode and Marcy Edelman, "Elderly Homosexual Women and Men: Report on a Pilot Study," *Family Coordinator*, Vol 27 (4), October 1978, pp. 451-456.

4. Chris Almvig, "The Invisible Minority: Aging and Lesbianism," Master's Thesis, April, 1982. Raymond M. Berger, "The Unseen Minority, Older Gays and Lesbians," *Social Work,* May, 1982, pp. 236-242.

5. Jim Kelly, "The Aging Male Homosexual: Myth and Reality," *The Gerontologist,* Vol 17, #41, 1977, pp. 328-333.

6. Kimmel, p. 120.

7. United Way awarded SAGE a grant of $32,000.

8. Community Board #2 Archive Fund awarded SAGE $18,000 and New York Community Trust awarded $20,000.

9. Gay Care Committee, "Fundraising in the Gay Community: A Perspective For 1982," Mimeo. San Francisco, 1982. (Available from the Gay Care Committee, P.O. Box 22612, San Francisco, California 94122.)

II

Life Problems

Confronting Homophobia
in Health Care Settings:
Guidelines for Social Work Practice

Alice E. Messing
Robert Schoenberg
Roger K. Stephens

There are special considerations in the provision of health care services to gay men and lesbians. Fear of gay men and lesbians and discrimination against them are major obstacles in the provision of health care services to this population.

Basic to social work practice is the perspective that social workers work at the intersection of society and the individual, attempting to achieve appropriate changes in both individuals and the society in which they live. Accordingly, social workers can play a vital role in improving health services for gay and lesbian patients by countering fear and discrimination—in themselves, in health care settings, and in patients.

HOMOPHOBIA

Homophobia is the irrational fear of love and affection between members of the same sex. Homophobia and the discrimination it produces permeate our society. Homophobia cripples all people similar to the way racism hurts whites as well as blacks, and the way anti-semitism can paralyze an entire society as well as the Jewish population in it (as in Germany in the 1930s).

The manifestations of homophobia are numerous. They include various stereotypes which are familiar to all of us through "fag jokes." Stereotypes continue in spite of the increasing public sophistication about gay men and lesbians resulting from the Gay

Liberation Movement and the Women's Liberation Movement. Although most social workers now know better than to believe that all lesbians are male-identified, and would laugh at the misconception that all gay men are limp-wristed, more subtle stereotypes have been more difficult to dispel. These include the myth that no gay men or lesbians are in heterosexual marriages, that all gay men have large expendable incomes, that gay men and lesbians are not interested in child-rearing, and that all gay men and lesbians are politically left of center. In reality, some gay men and lesbians *are* married, some gay men *are* in low income brackets, many gay men and lesbians *are* raising children, and a substantial number of gay men and lesbians *are* conservative on issues of economics and politics.

Estimates of the numbers of people who are gay are generally in the range of 5–10% of the population. Based on a conservative estimate and assuming a case load of twenty-five patients each month, in one year a social worker would have 15 gay patients. Yet many workers would be hard pressed to identify even five gay patients in the course of a career. It is difficult to believe that we know so little about our clients.

Denial is one of the primary manifestations of homophobia. Statistics about the large numbers of gay men and lesbians are often dismissed as exaggerations by the same individuals who falsely believe that the nuclear family is predominant. The role of gay men and lesbians in history has been denied also.

UNDERSTANDING HOMOPHOBIA IN SOCIAL WORKERS

Health care providers—just as all other people—are products of a culture and socialization process which are homophobic. Thus, there is a variety of provider reactions and attitudes regarding lesbian/gay sexual orientation. We assume that providers' attitudes and reactions are related to many factors, including their comfort with their own sexuality. We do not assume that lesbian/gay providers are inevitably accepting and understanding of lesbian/gay patients. This view reiterates our assumption that homophobia is a pervasive social condition, the results of which need to be recognized and counteracted. There is the possibility that lesbian or gay providers' work with lesbian or gay patients will be enhanced by strong identifications, though over-identification is also a possibility. A provider's reactions are not uniform; to some extent, they are situation-specific. It is important for health care providers to understand their reactions and attitudes and work to modify them when necessary and possible.

A common reaction among educated people with a liberal world view is that sexual orientation doesn't make any difference. Frequently we hear statements which begin, "It doesn't matter who one sleeps with...." This attitude ignores that for many lesbians and gay men, sexual orientation has had a profound impact on their lives which must be taken into account when providing social work services.

Hostility is another attitude found among workers. Open contempt for lesbians and gay men may result in the refusal to provide services or an attempt to convert lesbians and gay men to be heterosexual. A resident at a major teaching hospital told one of the authors that if an openly gay patient presented with a strep throat, he would also "treat" the patient's sexuality, prescribing the Bible along with antibiotics. To this physician, the cure for the strep throat was linked to a "cure" for the patient's gay identity.

Another type of reaction is exaggerating the significance of sexual orientation. In this case, more is made of the fact that a patient is gay or lesbian than is germane to the presenting problem. For example, a patient was grieving the loss of a parent in an automobile accident. An intern read in the medical record that the patient was gay and noticed that he was depressed. The intern immediately began to "counsel" the patient to the effect that being gay was the cause of his depression.

Denial of sexuality is an all-too-common reaction, especially with regard to older people who are the most frequent consumers of health care services. As a result, social workers, along with other health care providers, are often blind to significant information which patients are willing to share. For example, when a social worker interviewed an older man regarding a discharge plan, she asked about how his wife would manage his care. When he responded that he did not have a wife, the worker immediately assumed that he lived alone. It was later that she learned of his life-long "friend" who became the care-giver.

Some social workers see homosexuality as a problem and a burden and therefore react by taking pity on gay men and lesbians. Fortunately, various liberation movements have done much to counter these attitudes.

Another provider response is admiration. This view recognizes the accomplishments made by some lesbians and gay men despite discrimination and against great odds.

COUNTERING HOMOPHOBIA IN SOCIAL WORKERS

We might hope that all social workers would respond to lesbians and gay men in an informed, sensitive manner, with an understanding of their own reactions and attitudes (as well as with an appreciation of the personal histories of the patients, especially as they relate to health care). However, as indicated by the range of reactions and attitudes just described, it is necessary for most social workers to confront some manifestations of homophobia in themselves. Homophobia can be confronted in at least three ways: (1) exploring one's own history, (2) learning the facts, and (3) getting to know lesbians and gay men.

In exploring the roots of homophobia, it is necessary to consider cultural and personal history. Social workers should think about their early attitudes toward lesbians and gay men; remember the first lesbian or gay man they saw/talked with/were friends with/loved. Social workers should ask themselves what labels they used for lesbians and gay men when they were growing up. Do they have any lesbian or gay friends now? They should get in touch with their feelings about same-sex affection and eroticism and begin to overcome their internal barriers.

Learning the facts is certainly much easier today than even ten years ago. Many excellent books have been written which can be resources for the social worker wanting to learn more about the issues, concerns, and feelings of lesbians and gay men (Gay Task Force, American Library Association, 1980).

Research has shown that those who know lesbians and gay men personally are less likely to have fears and misunderstandings about them (Hansen, 1982). There are many opportunities to meet, talk with, and listen to lesbians and gay men. These include going to a lesbian or gay movie, concert, or cultural event, visiting a lesbian/gay bookstore, participating in a lesbian/gay rights meeting, march or demonstration. These opportunities are an invaluable resource for confronting one's homophobia and preparing for confronting homophobia in health care settings.

UNDERSTANDING INTERNALIZED HOMOPHOBIA IN PATIENTS

Gay men and lesbians have been brought up in the same culture and environment we have been discussing. Thus, they have been exposed to and may have internalized the same homophobia. It is important for social workers to recognize manifestations of internalized homophobia.

Lesbians and gay men often experience particular anxiety or guilt about having a health problem. There are historical roots for this. Homosexuality was first categorized as a disease by nineteenth century physicians, and health professionals generally have held that view until recently. It is not surprising that some lesbians and gay men irrationally feel that a physical illness is caused by their sexual orientation.

The recent AIDS* outbreak has provoked a virtual panic reaction among the gay male subculture. Under the circumstances, a certain amount of apprehension could be expected. But the reactions of many go far beyond that: some men are renouncing sexual behavior which has not been implicated in the cause of AIDS, while others are taking the diseases as a cause for condemnation of their sexual orientation. The readiness of some gay men to be self-punitive exposes the extensive damage of internalized homophobia.

WHAT SOCIAL WORKERS CAN DO ABOUT HOMOPHOBIA

Having acknowledged the existence of homophobia in providers, in patients, and in health care settings, it is important to identify what social workers can do about homophobia. Social workers in health care settings must be sensitive to the experiences of lesbians and gay men in order to understand reluctance to engage in treatment and hostility to health care. The social worker has a number of important specific contributions to make in the health

---

*Acquired immune deficiency syndrome involves the breakdown of the immune system, the body's defense against disease. This renders victims vulnerable to "opportunistic" infections such as Kaposi's Sarcoma, and Pneumocystis Carinii Pneumonia. Most, but not all, victims of AIDS have been gay men.

care of a lesbian or gay patient: as a translator or communication link between a patient and the medical staff, as the patient's advocate in a frequently hostile environment, as a health educator for both the patient and the medical team, and as a developer of new services.

COMMUNICATION LINK

Open communication between provider and patient is key to the delivery of high quality health care. The patient who does not have access to empathetic and understanding health care providers will be uncomfortable relating all kinds of medically relevant information or may avoid contact with the health care system.

A social worker can facilitate communication between patients and other providers. Often, the lesbian or gay patient needs to be encouraged and supported to relate pertinent information about the transmission of a disease or patterns of health to the provider. And recognizing that the physician's successful diagnosis and treatment may be dependent on his or her ability to elicit and comprehend sensitive information, the social worker can help physicians who have a lack of experience with lesbians and gay men to use sensitive language, ask pertinent questions, and overcome their initial discomfort working with an unfamiliar patient group.

The social worker may be a referral source or in other ways help a patient select the best medical practitioner. For example, the patient needs to be counseled that although the practitioner's comfort in discussing the patient's sexuality is important, such communication should not be sought at the expense of competency. Switching physicians is often problematic. First, there are no sure ways of identifying competent and receptive providers and, second, multiple initial office visits are costly. Especially in a medical crisis, the social worker may have a responsibility to help a patient and physician overcome communication barriers and to continue to work together. Consider, for example, the challenges involved when a gay or lesbian patient is admitted through an emergency room and the case is assigned to an extremely homophobic or hostile physician. It is taxing enough on a patient to have to explain his or her life style while well, but while contending with illness it can become impossible. Thus the role of the social worker to understand and advocate on behalf of the patient becomes clear.

ADVOCATE

Conflicts between the needs of physicians, hospital administrators, other members of the health care team and the patient make for a confusing situation. The social worker must be prepared to go to bat for the patient and to support the patient's interests. At times, advocacy precludes encouraging the patient to come out while defenses are lower due to illness. At other times, it may mean encouraging a patient to come out to the physician, especially if a sexually transmitted disease is suspected or when the conflicts of trying to remain closeted are too great.

The worker can provide assistance so that the patient receives necessary care. This may include supporting the patient's right to have a partner visit in the hospital even if the relationship makes some members of the hospital staff uncomfortable. A patient may choose to have a close friend or partner make crucial medical decisions on his or her behalf, instead of a parent or other blood relative. A social worker in that situation should support the patient's wishes and may help the excluded relative understand why. Helping the patient may require the social worker to overcome his or her prejudices and not to project his or her personal values on the patient. Many times a patient will not be clear in expressing the need to have gay friends or a partner in the hospital. This may be motivated by fear of rejection by hospital staff and providers. In this case, the social worker must recognize the importance of a patient's access to his or her personal support network in the recovery process. It may be essential to involve the person with whom the patient lives in the care of the patient after being discharged. The social worker may need to encourage gay or lesbian patients to allow the people who are closest in life to call, visit, and send gifts.

Supporting a patient's right to self-determination is an important part of patient advocacy. Self-determination is an essential element of social work practice and must be maintained vigorously in working with lesbian and gay patients. For example, an inexperienced worker wrote a note in the medical chart which indicated that the patient was gay. When the patient learned of the note, he became very upset and angry, demanding that it be removed from the record. The patient's statement "I will come out to whom I chose and when I chose" reflects his need for self-determination. The worker rightly felt that the patient's homosexuality was relevant to his health care. Unfortunately, the worker failed to engage the patient in the process of determining his health care. The consequences to the patient could have been dramatic. Employers can gain access to medical records for insurance purposes and careers can be jeopardized. Relationships with hospital staff and relatives may be disrupted. Some staff may avoid caring for the patient while others may try to "convert" the patient.

Inexperienced workers may be overly anxious to find out if the patient is gay or they may be totally insensitive to patients' attempts to tell of their significant relationships. Directness in asking the patient is not always called for. One valuable source of information is the admission or intake sheet. It should be a matter of habit to notice the patient's marital status and who is listed as nearest relative or "significant other." It is important that admission data be collected accurately and clearly as well as in a way that will avoid possible negative consequences for the patient. For example, in some facilities admission forms ask for "person to contact in emergency" rather than "spouse" thus allowing for more flexibility on the part of the patient. A social worker may encourage a lesbian or gay man to consider a power of attorney to authorize someone other than a blood relative to make crucial medical decisions if the patient is unable to make them for himself or herself and to entitle that person to the same hospital privileges customarily granted to a member of the patient's family. In addition to visitation rights, and the right to give or withhold consent about medical decisions, the power of attorney along with a will may provide help in case of death, by delegating the right to personal effects and decisions about the disposal of the body to a non-family member. Using available data allows health providers to frame questions about relationships without forcing the patient to be dishonest about sexual orientation or to disclose more than he or she wishes to disclose. Thus, patients need to be informed about their rights and the possible consequences of revealing or not revealing certain information so that they can truly determine for themselves.

EDUCATOR

A host of health problems can be greatly reduced and eventually eradicated through proper health education programs which are non-judgmental, targeted to the appropriate populations, and promote the concept that self-knowledge is important. Such programs would help, for example, the lesbian who avoids routine pelvic examinations and pap tests, erroneously believing that only heterosexually active women need to be concerned about cervical cancer, and the gay man who has sexual relations when he has hepatitis not knowing that it is possible that he can give the disease to his partner. Social workers can also educate the medical community. They can share what they have learned in working with gay men and lesbians and they can encourage health professionals to familiarize themselves with the growing body of literature about gay/lesbian health and the relevance of sexual orientation to the provision of health care.

In many public schools, young people are taught about birth control and prevention of venereal diseases for those who are heterosexually active; but homosexuality is usually not mentioned and the health care needs of lesbians and gay men are ignored. Students need to be forewarned that the symptoms of gonorrhea and syphilis may not be apparent in the rectum and throat, but that a simple test can be used to diagnose the presence or absence of these diseases. Young women who are desirous of having children need to be informed that artificial insemination is a legitimate alternative to heterosexual intercourse as a means of becoming pregnant. Some lesbians and gay men are fearful of coming out to their health care providers and many health care providers are ignorant of what advice to give to lesbian and gay patients. Thus, most lesbians and gay males grow up at risk of acquiring diseases and experiencing other health problems about which their families, schools, and the medical establishment have provided inadequate information.

Given the lack of information about lesbian and gay health and the discomfort about sexual issues in general even among health professionals, it is not uncommon for some patients to feel excessively upset about having even a common and easily treated sexually transmitted disease. Social work educators and counselors have an important role in relieving lesbians and gay men of inappropriate guilt about these matters. For example, Philadelphia Community Health Alternatives, a non-profit corporation specializing in meeting the health care needs of sexual minorities, utilizes social workers at its venereal disease clinic to help dispel the patient's guilt, to reinforce the patient's understanding of the germ theory of disease, and to refer a patient with religious concerns to an enlightened religious counselor. Social workers, along with nurse educators, offer practical advice about how a sexually active individual can reduce the risk of acquiring infectious diseases through proper diet, adequate sleep, and hygienic practices.

SERVICE DEVELOPER

Social workers can take the lead as institution builders as well as being educational reformers. Indeed, social workers have a long and proud history of originating innovative social service agencies to meet new and changing social needs. In response to the gap in qualified health services for lesbians and gay men, concerned professionals worked together to establish lesbian and gay health centers in most major metropolitan areas. These centers provide sensitive and competent health services and referrals. Social workers with community organizing experience can help establish such centers where they don't already exist and help maintain ones where they do.

CONCLUSION

A practice based on striving to eradicate homophobia is consistent with core social work values as embodied in the Code of Ethics and elsewhere. Participating in the provision of health services to lesbians and gay men also offers social workers an excellent opportunity to put essential social work principles into practice. In countering an oppressive force and in providing quality services, these social workers are engaging in exemplary social work practice.

SELECTED REFERENCE LIST

Curry, H. and Clifford, D. *A Legal Guide for Lesbian and Gay Couples.* Reading, MA: Addison Wesley, 1980.

Dardick, L. and Grady, K. E. Openness Between Gay Persons and Health Professionals. *Annals of Internal Medicine,* 1980, *93* (Part 1), 115-119.

Gay Task Force, American Library Association. *A Gay Bibliography, 6th Edition.* Philadelphia, PA: Gay Task Force, American Library Association (Social Responsibilities Round Table), March 1980. (Gay Task Force of ALA, P.O. Box 2383, Philadelphia, PA 19103).

Hansen, G. L. Measuring Prejudice Against Homosexuality (Homosexism) Among College Students: A New Scale. *The Journal of Social Psychology,* 1982, *117,* 233-236.

Homosexuality and Alcoholism:
Social and Developmental Perspectives

Marta Ann Zehner
Joyce Lewis

"Among the gay and lesbian population probably 20%–30% are alcoholic, twice to three times as large a percentage as in the general population."[1] Thus, there is compelling reason to examine the relationship between homosexuality and alcoholism. That is the primary purpose of this article.

The article is divided into three areas: a general description and definition of alcoholism as a problem in our society; special issues for gays and lesbians and their vulnerability to alcoholism; services for alcoholics generally and services geared specifically to lesbian and gay alcoholics.

ALCOHOLISM AND OUR SOCIETY

Although the use of marijuana is still widespread among teenagers as well as older people, alcohol is becoming the number one drug for the very young. A survey done by the NIAAA (National Institute on Alcohol Abuse and Alcoholism, U.S. Dept. of HEW) in 1978, reported that 62% of 7th graders and 80% of 8th graders drank.[2] It is not uncommon for 16 and 17 year old people to join Alcoholics Anonymous. Using conventional estimates regarding the occurrence of homosexuality in the general population, it is likely that at least 10% of these teenagers are gay and lesbian.

The estimated 9 million alcoholics in the U.S. represent a wide cross section of American life: students, plumbers, real estate agents, physicians, housewives, writers, painters, clergy, farmers, stock brokers, academics, secretaries, fifteen year-olds and folks in their seventies. Every ethnic group, religious denomination and social class is represented. Stereotypical skid row bums, representing only 3% of the alcoholic population, are simply people from the other categories whose drinking has taken them to jobless, homeless lives of panhandling for survival. Most alcoholics find their own personal skid row in the neighborhood bar or in their own kitchen, living room or bedroom.

Alcoholism ranks as one of the major causes of death, claiming more victims than any other illnesses except heart disease and cancer. The life expectancy of the alcoholic is 10–12 years shorter than the non-alcoholic. According to research conducted by The National Council on Alcoholism, a national voluntary organization which sponsors research, evaluation, prevention and education in the field of alcoholism, diagnosis on admission to a general hospital frequently omits alcohol as a factor in the illness; in fact, excessive use of alcohol is often a significant part of the picture in diseases of the circulatory, digestive, respiratory, nervous and endocrine systems. In addition, alcohol plays a part in a significant percentage of accidental and violent deaths. The National Council on Alcoholism, also has found that alcohol contributes to 50% of all highway deaths, 47% of non-fatal industrial accidents, 40% of fatal industrial accidents, 83% of fire fatalities, 62% of burns, 70% of deaths from falls, 63% of injuries from falls. In one of our major cities, the director of the county alcoholism program reports that alcohol is present as a significant factor in 64% of homicides, 56% of domestic fights or assaults, 71% of accidental poisonings, 72% of beatings, 30% of suicides, and 67% of sexually aggressive acts against children. The cost of alcoholism to business and industry nationwide is $19 billion annually.[3]

According to the National Council on Alcoholism, there are 90,000,000 persons in the U.S. who drink alcohol. Many of those people enjoy alcohol as a social lubricant or as a source of relaxation on infrequent occasions. Some others use it on a daily basis and encounter no problem in their lives on account of its use. Among those 90,000,000, there are 9,000,000 (a conservative estimate) who have crossed an invisible line and are alcoholic.[4] Many of these 9,000,000 are addicted to at least one other substance, including the ubiquitous cigarette.

The causes of alcoholism are probably several and the etiology (predisposition, learned behavior, etc.) remains open. Experts in the field disagree as to whether or not alcoholism can be called a "disease," though no one disagrees that treatment is indicated;

health insurance plans provide coverage for that treatment. Regardless of cause, alcoholism usually follows a specific course. Though the first drink(s) may be taken on a social occasion, the feelings experienced (euphoria, lessening of anxiety, loss of social inhibition) have a profound effect on the potential alcoholic. In fact, even on the first occasion of drinking, the pleasant feelings may lead to excessive drinking, drunkenness and blackout (temporary memory loss). The alcoholic quickly develops tolerance for large amounts of alcohol without showing signs of drunkenness and frequently is the person who drives everyone else home from the party. Consumption gradually increases as the body requires more of the drug to produce the same effect. One sign of trouble is the person's inability to limit himself/herself to a predetermined amount of alcohol or to determine the occasions on which he/she drinks. As drinking increases, physical problems may develop and certainly the general level of health is affected. At some point, physiological and psychological dependence on the drug is established. Because an acceptable level of comfort is only possible through the ingestion of ethyl alcohol, the alcoholic continues to drink, regardless of the consequences. And they are many. All areas of the person's life are affected adversely, including the social, physical, psychological, spiritual and vocational. Alcohol is now the focus of the person's attention: getting it, drinking it, hiding it, recovering from the effects of it, making excuses for behavior while under the influence of it. By now, friends, family and employer are probably aware of the problem and if, by chance, they have the audacity to suggest that the alcoholic is drinking too much, they are likely to hear one of the following: 1) "I can stop whenever I want to," 2) "I've only had a couple," 3) "Maybe I should change from martinis to wine or beer," 4) "You'd drink too, if you had my lover, (boss, parents, teacher, job, problems, etc.)." Those responses point to two of the defense mechanisms commonly used by alcoholics (though not exclusively by alcoholics), namely denial and projection. Unfortunately, people who are close to the alcoholic often accept the excuses and the promises. And alcohol-dependent people continue to minimize the problem as well as place responsibility on everything and everyone for their failures. Unless intervention occurs at this point, the course of the disease is usually downhill to physical debilitation, disruption of social relationships, unemployment, major organic mental illness (Wernicke's syndrome, Korsakoff's syndrome) or death. This process—from the first drink to irreversible physical and mental catastrophe—may take many years. One thing seems clear: that if the alcoholic continues to drink, his/her social, emotional, physical life will deteriorate. At the very least the active alcoholic functions at only 50–60% of his/her potential.

Alcohol and other drugs are used to produce pleasant effects and, for those who become addicted, to avoid temporarily the difficulties of life. One only has to watch the ads on television for a very short time to get the message that if you have any discomfort or pain there is 1) something wrong with you and 2) a ready, easily obtainable solution is available in the form of a pill, liquid, salve, or spray to remove the symptom. Life is not supposed to be difficult. Although there are other time-tested ways to relax and have a good time, alcohol is the most commonly used drug for this purpose on many social occasions. When was the last time you attended a dinner party at which alcohol was not served? Or a wedding, funeral, bar mitzvah, birthday, retirement, back-to-work party, etc.? Most people can safely drink alcohol and limit the amount. The alcoholic cannot. The relationship between the person and the drug loses the quality of choice and that relationship becomes primary. Obsession with the drug of choice and compulsion to use it take precedence over other matters in the addicted person's life. Interest is withdrawn from other aspects of life although a facade of "normal" activity may be presented.

THE LESBIAN AND GAY COMMUNITY AND ALCOHOL

Having discussed alcoholism in general this paper will now address issues regarding homosexuality and alcoholism. While we do not believe that there is any causal relationship between homosexuality and alcoholism, we do believe that it is important to understand some of the inherent stresses, issues and patterns which may contribute to some lesbians' and gay men's vulnerability to alcoholism.

After working for a number of years with gay men and, in particular, lesbians, one of the authors (Zehner) began to identify what she thought of as patterns in the development of a lesbian/gay identity. The patterns are based on three variables: individual personality, the inherent oppression toward homosexuality in the larger society, the availability of a lesbian/gay community and support system. Six phases have been identified in the development of a lesbian/gay identity. We will use a discussion of these stages to identify common stresses for lesbians and gay men, how those stresses relate to alcohol use and alcoholism, and how the lesbian/gay community can either support alcoholism in its members or offer alternatives to excessive alcohol use and alcoholism. The six phases are: recognition, denial, confusion, fear, pride, integration.

Before describing in detail the 6 stages in the development of the lesbian/gay identity, it is important to note that these stages may or may not be sequential, each may last for years, months or a shorter period of time, and individuals may move back and forth among the various stages, depending upon the degree of stress, support, and other issues existing in their lives at any given time.

The first stage is the recognition that one is different than others in one's feelings and experiences toward people of the same sex. This recognition generally causes some confusion and anxiety, particularly since the individual somehow senses that this experience is not generally acceptable. S/he usually chooses not to discuss this with anyone else, and it is common for the individual to move into the next stage, which is an attempt at denial.

In the attempt at denial, the individual usually works hard to feel and behave just like everyone else in the larger society, particularly peers. S/he becomes skilled at imitation. There may be a great flurry of heterosexual activity and attempts (successful or not successful) to form meaningful relationships with people of the opposite sex. There is an attempt to put out of one's awareness the confusing feeling toward the same sex and this often causes tension within the individual. It is in this stage that many people have entered therapy, hoping to change themselves enough to become heterosexual, and rid themselves of the underlying tension.

Joe was 20 and a college junior when he sought psychiatric help for his homosexuality. He told the psychiatrist that he wanted to become heterosexual, that the pain of being homosexual, not fitting in, being lonely and feeling isolated, was too much to bear. For two years, Joe received positive feedback from his psychiatrist when he dated women and negative feedback when he gave into the urge to date another man. During this period of time, his consumption of alcohol increased greatly. As graduation drew nearer, he realized that he was no closer to being heterosexual.

Joe's experience is not an unusual one. Never during the course of his therapy did Joe's psychiatrist explore with him his feelings about homosexuality, his factual knowledge of homosexuality, of other homosexuals and the gay culture, or his support system within the gay community. Joe's psychiatrist automatically accepted Joe's simplistic analysis of the problem: "Since I'm unhappy as a homosexual I should try to become heterosexual." There are few, if any, other issues in which a mental health practitioner would so easily support a client's unrealistic wish, rather than assist the individual in finding a deeper understanding of his/her feelings, behavior, and alternatives for life choices. The issues for Joe were his lack of understanding of homosexuality, his lack of connection to other gay men and hence his feelings of loneliness and isolation, his internalized oppression, the beliefs that homosexuality is bad, wrong, sick, and immoral. With an exploration of these issues and support to do so, Joe could have been freed up emotionally to see that he did have various choices for seeking personal fulfillment. The increase in Joe's alcohol consumption was never addressed in his therapy either. Joe became increasingly aware of using alcohol to help him survive a date with a woman and to help him block out his guilty feelings after a date with a man. The alcohol was serving to numb more and more of Joe's experience of himself as it also interfered with his everyday functioning and endangered his life. The psychiatrist was focused on changing Joe's sexual-affectional feelings and viewed his homosexuality and alcoholic behavior as secondary. In fact, in this instance, homosexuality and alcohol behavior were not causally related, but needed to be addressed simultaneously. Joe should have been helped to confront and understand his feelings of homosexuality and offered alternatives for how to explore its meaning in his life. He also needed to confront his use of alcohol and understand this as a sign that he would continue to misuse alcohol in his life unless he made another decision. He needed to understand this not as an isolated time in his life when he drank too much but as a warning signal that he is vulnerable to alcoholism.

Social workers and other mental health practitioners have often mistreated both alcoholism and homosexuality. This mistreatment has often been a result of lack of information and sometimes of a value judgment against those who were alcoholic, homosexual, or both. If a lesbian or gay man requested treatment for depression or unhappiness in a relationship, the professional often attempted to change the client's sexual orientation, assuming that this would clear up the depression. Most attempts were unsuccessful and many health professionals have now learned that this is inappropriate. The homosexuality was treated as a disease instead of recognizing that the internalized oppression was at the core of the depression. It is this fact that still causes many lesbian and gay men to hesitate to seek professional counseling.

Social workers and other mental health professionals have also not understood alcoholism as a disease and have not known how to treat it. In the past, alcoholics have been engaged by helping professionals in searches for the underlying psychic causes while they continued to drink themselves to death. It was not understood that the first step to treating alcoholism is recognizing it as a disease and helping the alcoholic give up alcohol.

Lesbian/gay alcoholics seeking treatment have lived with a double jeopardy: ignorance on the part of professionals about both alcoholism and homosexuality. Lesbian/gay alcoholics must always be treated directly for alcoholism while being assisted in uprooting the internalized oppression and in finding ways to accept themselves as worthy people.

The third phase in the development of a lesbian/gay identity is confusion. When individuals can no longer deny the feeling of homosexuality, they usually experience a great deal of confusion and anxiety. They realize that this frightening part of themselves must be faced but do not know how. Who should they talk to? Who will listen without judging? Where can they go to get information, meet others, and create opportunities to become more familiar with this part of themselves. Since most people can tolerate high levels of anxiety and confusion for only limited periods of time, this phase usually ends with the decision to repress feelings of homosexuality or to acknowledge the feelings and explore the meaning, the lifestyles or the choices available to those who wish to understand more about their homosexuality.

But, of course, another way to deal with the confusion and anxiety is to use excessive amounts of alcohol or any other drug to block out these uncomfortable feelings. The alcohol deadens the anxiety and confusion, thus bringing temporary relief to the individual; but when the effects of the alcohol wear off, the anxiety and confusion return, creating the need to use something to again deaden the sensations of anxiety and confusion. The emotional and the physiological need for the alcohol increases and the cycle of alcoholism begins. Providing help to people caught in this cycle presents a dilemma: they cannot make effective use of counseling while using alcohol excessively to anesthetize their feelings, yet giving up the alcohol and confronting these feelings seems too painful. Giving up the alcohol is the first step and the counselor must be prepared for the intense anxiety and discomfort that will immediately follow and have resources available to help the client through this difficult period. These resources can include, among others, the use of support people and/or support groups, techniques for relaxation and managing anxiety, and a conceptual framework for understanding questions and confusion about homosexuality. If these and other resources are not available, or if the individuals do not make use of them, then they are at greater risk for returning to drinking.

The next phase which involves the beginning acknowledgment and acceptance of one's homosexuality is usually characterized by extreme fear that others will discover this secret. Individuals often become overly secretive, highly anxious, and even angry that so much of their energy must be spent in covering up their homosexuality. The fear is that if others find out about their homosexuality, their jobs, family relationships and friendships will be at risk. And for many lesbians and gay men, this is a realistic fear.

Individuals may choose to read books to gain more information about homosexuality, or may enter therapy to understand more about their own feelings and desires. They may start attending functions in the lesbian/gay community and may begin relating to other lesbians and gay men. They may use lesbian/gay support groups to examine if, how and when they want to share this personal information about themselves with close friends and family. Any and all of these can be important to people in their growing need to understand and accept their homosexuality.

> Laura is a 35 year old single woman, living with another woman in a lesbian relationship. She teaches at a local community college where she has been employed for many years. She presented herself for therapy with the complaint of severe anxiety attacks which interfered with her ability to

teach, mix in groups of people or attend social functions. In further discussion it became clear that Laura was uncomfortable with her lesbianism, felt forced to hide her lifestyle from colleagues, family and friends; as a result she felt angry and isolated. As her feelings about her homosexuality were explored, it became clear that she was torn between believing that her lifestyle was okay and feeling that it was wrong and sinful. She had been a religious woman and her experience with her church's position on homosexuality substantiated her belief that she was living a sinful, immoral life. Her fear and isolation from the lesbian community kept her from seeing any positive lesbian role models, and she felt trapped in her lesbianism. While taking a routine drinking history, it also became apparent that she was drinking excessively.

While Laura came to therapy concerned about her anxiety attacks and while it was also apparent that there were many other problems, the starting point had to be dealing with her alcoholism. None of the other problems could be adequately assessed while Laura was actively drinking. After Laura was connected with a local Alcoholics Anonymous group and was assisted in confronting the beginning steps of her alcoholism, she was ready to examine the attitudes and beliefs about her lesbianism that she had internalized. This involved Laura's willingness to uncover her own myths and stereotypes about lesbians as well as her deep seated belief that being homosexual indicated there was something intrinsically wrong with her. Laura was also directed to use the lesbian/gay resources in her community to reeducate herself and place her in contact with lesbian and gay people who were proud of their sexual identity.

A particular obstacle encountered in the lesbian/gay community is that the lesbian/gay bar or club is often the pivotal social institution. Frequently, it is to the bar that people go in the hope of meeting someone new or some old friends, to celebrate birthdays, major holidays, to pass time, or to create the illusion of not being alone. The bar is often seen as, and often is, the only social institution in a community specifically for lesbian and gay people. It is here that lesbians and gays do not need to worry about feeling different or being accepted. They can look around them and see a room filled with other lesbians and/or gay men, and if, perchance, there are heterosexual persons present, they are definitely in the minority and also not likely to be critical. This makes the bar a comfortable place for lesbians and gay men. Here they can be themselves and not fear being stigmatized or ostracized. The need for this safety cannot be minimized. Every minority culture builds institutions to celebrate its uniqueness. The gathering together helps to lessen the feelings of isolation. It is in many ways unfortunate that the bar has become the most recognized institution in the lesbian/gay culture because along with it comes the tradition of using alcohol while socializing and as the main psychic relief.

Since the lesbian/gay bar is often the most recognized social institution in the lesbian/gay community, the social worker must be ready to assist lesbian/gay clients, particularly those with drinking problems, to identify alternatives. In many lesbian/gay communities, there are alternatives. A lesbian/gay community center may provide support through social, educational and recreational activities. There are lesbian/gay churches and synagogues which provide spiritual comfort, social activities, and acceptance to many lesbian/gay people. There are lesbian/gay bookstores, restaurants, health care facilities, and counseling centers, as well as social networks which provide opportunities to meet other lesbian/gay people in social settings apart from the bar scene. Women's concerts are used as a gathering for lesbians and supportive heterosexual women to pass on a lesbian art form and celebrate the lesbian identity in a supportive environment. It is critical for social workers working with lesbian/gay clients to learn about the lesbian/gay facilities in their communities and to encourage clients to socialize, celebrate, and find comfort in their identity with lesbians and gay men in places other than bars.

As lesbian/gay individuals in this phase of development move more into the lesbian/gay community, they have to learn how to negotiate two different worlds. They determine to what extent they will participate in the lesbian/gay culture and in the larger heterosexual culture. There are those lesbians and gay men who choose to live as completely as possible in the lesbian/gay subculture. While this may seem to provide more protection from the stress of dealing in the larger heterosexual culture, it also has the effect of emphasizing the oppression that homosexuals feel since they become so much more conscious of having to live separately in order to maintain a sense of acceptability.

On the other hand, to choose to negotiate these two different worlds adds another dimension of potential stress for lesbians and gay men. There are those lesbians and gay men who participate more in the larger heterosexual culture and are constantly aware of how unacceptable homosexuality is in the larger American culture. They live in constant fear that someone will discover their lesbianism/homosexuality and the resulting stress makes some of the more vulnerable to alcohol misuse and alcoholism. Once again, it is important to stress alcoholism must be addressed and treated directly. It is also important to understand with clients' their acceptance or non-acceptance of their lifestyle. Among lesbians and gay men who are alcoholic, there are those for whom their homosexuality is not in any way related to their drinking. It is inappropriate then to focus on a connection between sexual-affectional orientation and their alcoholism.

People who have moved into the next phase are lesbian/gay and proud of it. Here, the lesbian or gay man is no longer fearful that others will discover his/her homosexuality. Lesbian and gay men, at this point, have usually found role models, participated fully in the lesbian/gay community, and are proud of their homosexuality. These are the individuals who have already evaluated or faced the risk of losing jobs, family and friendships. Some of them have experienced deep losses as a result of that risk and must look to the lesbian/gay community as their primary support system. Every oppressed group needs leaders and front-line fighters. In the lesbian/gay movement, many of those leaders and fighters come from those who are in this phase in the development of their identity. This is the time when individuals assert their power in positive ways to fight both the oppression of the external world and the internalized oppression they have been enduring. Though these individuals may have found support in the lesbian/gay community, they still need to negotiate the larger society. Sometimes the differences in the experiences they have in the lesbian/gay community and the larger society create anger and discontentment. This can be a good excuse for drinking, particularly if the individual is vulnerable to using alcohol to handle uncomfortable feelings. A well-informed and sensitive social worker understands the burden that front-line lesbian/gay clients may be carrying and does not help them use it as justification for excessive use of alcohol.

The sixth and final phase is integration. Integration represents individuals having acknowledged and accepted homosexuality and worked through a lot of the internalized oppression. They have reached a high level of openness in relationships and in the world and are therefore free to experience homosexuality as an integral part of themselves but not as the only aspect of their identity.

It is useful for social workers to understand that each of these phases is important to lesbians and gay men in developing the sense of identity they need in order to survive in the larger society. Lesbians and gay men must be supported wherever they are in the process of developing this identity. Mental health professionals must understand the pain involved in confronting one's difference and the disapproval from the outside world as well as the pride and power which result from accepting and asserting that difference.

We have described in detail developmental and social issues for gays and lesbians, believing that the social worker who understands these issues will work more effectively with gay men and lesbians who are alcoholic. However, in working with gay men and lesbians who are alcoholic, the social worker must always focus on the alcoholism and be clear that the first step is to help clients give up the alcohol. Gay and lesbian clients, like all clients, will respect and trust the social worker if they sense that the social worker understands the particular issues that are problematic and painful for them. Many gay men and lesbians who are alcoholic and looking for help with this problem are hesitant to contact a counselor or alcohol facility for fear of rejection, humiliation, or lack of understanding about homosexuality. Therefore, it is important for counselors to be both knowledgeable and sensitive about special issues for gay and lesbian alcoholics.

ALCOHOLISM SERVICES

There is a wide range of services available for the treatment of alcoholism. The number of services will vary depending on the particular community and it is the responsibility of social workers and other mental health professionals to be well acquainted with alcohol services in their community. Most programs welcome inquiries and extend themselves to provide information and education to other professionals.

The National Council on Alcoholism (NCA) is a voluntary organization that operates nationwide. NCA works toward the prevention and control of alcoholism. It works with local councils to offer information and referral services to alcoholics and their significant others. Many of these local councils also provide counseling. Community Mental Health Centers are mandated to provide alcoholism services to those living in their catchment area. The services provided by these centers will vary but most have outpatient services staffed by alcoholism counselors.

Public and general hospitals maintain detoxification units in order to detoxify those alcoholics whose withdrawal from ethyl alcohol could be problematic. Some private hospitals also maintain detoxification units. There are many residential treatment programs which provide intensive counseling, resocialization and education to alcoholics. These centers usually offer some outpatient treatment to the significant others involved with the alcoholic. There are often other public and private alcohol services in communities; the local health department or Alcohol Information Center can provide a list and description of services.

In recent years, business and industry have recognized the problem of alcoholism and have initiated employee programs. These programs involve the training of supervisors to recognize the signs of alcoholism and refer the employee to a confidential counseling service. The action of the supervisor is based on observation of poor or impaired job performance. The business may have its own counseling department or may have a contract with an agency in the community. In either case, the alcoholic employee is usually given the choice of going for help or being terminated. The American Medical Association long ago recognized alcoholism as a disease and Blue Cross-Blue Shield as well as other health plans provide coverage for its treatment. Many alcoholic employees are sent for detoxification and rehabilitation in one of the many programs across the country through their company health plans.

Continuing treatment following rehabilitation is necessary for the alcoholic and most programs refer the individual to Alcoholics Anonymous, the most successful treatment thus far. Many alcoholics recover through the use of A.A. without inpatient treatment in a rehabilitation center or any other treatment. Alcoholics Anonymous was started in 1935, in Akron, Ohio, by a stockbroker and a medical doctor, both "hopeless" alcoholics who had been treated by all the experts, unsuccessfully. At the present time, A.A. has groups all over the U.S. and in many foreign countries. Alcoholics Anonymous describes itself as a fellowship in which members "share their experience, strength and hope with each other that they may solve their common problem and help others to recover from alcoholism." The only requirement for membership is a desire to stop drinking. Once in A.A. the alcoholics begin to lose the sense of isolation which they have felt and begin to hear other members' experiences in solving problems without the use of alcohol or other drugs, through the use of the twelve steps which form the basis for recovery in A.A. These steps involve acknowledging dependence on alcohol and the disastrous effects of the misuse of alcohol on one's life and relationships with others. The support of the group is one of the most effective tools in recovery. Over 1.5 million persons worldwide are now recovering in A.A.

Large cities all over the U.S. now have meetings specifically for gay people. At a recent gay A.A. conference attended by one of the authors, an announcement was made that approval had been given for the development of literature for gay alcoholics.[5]

At meetings for lesbians and gay men, participants are able to speak freely about matters which are troubling to them and which might lead to drinking or drug use if not talked about in an accepting atmosphere. At a meeting of gay or lesbian alcoholics there is no need to be cautious about pronouns when referring to partners. Of course, lesbian and gay people attend other meetings of A.A. though they may omit references to same sex partners. If lesbian/gay alcoholics attend only meetings open to all alcoholics, their sharing (which is so much a part of the A.A. treatment process) may be limited; this can also diminish the effectiveness of the treatment. Individuals must choose which options they feel will be most helpful at any given time in the treatment process.

An outgrowth of Alcoholics Anonymous is the Al-Anon Family Group whose purpose is to provide hope and support to the families, loved ones, and friends of the alcoholic. Now there are also Gay Al-Anon meetings. These groups function according to the same general A.A. principles.

There has been an increase in professional literature concerning alcoholism and homosexuality, as well as the formation of a specialized professional organization, The National Association of Gay Alcoholism Professionals.[6] There continues to be the need for educating gay/lesbian alcoholics, alcohol professionals, and the general community about specific issues and needs of gay/lesbian alcoholics. NAGAP's goals are directed toward this end. The more that NAGAP and others are able to break through the negative stereotypes and misunderstandings that exist about both homosexuality and alcoholism, the greater the chance to provide help to gay and lesbian alcoholics and to develop successful strategies for prevention.

REFERENCES

1. Ziebold, Thomas O. "Alcoholism & Recovery: Gays Helping Gays," *Christopher Street*, January, 1979.

2. National Institute on Alcohol Abuse and Alcoholism, *The Answer Book*, U.S. Dept. of Health, Education and Welfare, Government Printing Office, 1978.

3. Riggs, Carol R. "Alcoholism—A $19 Billion Problem." Dunn and Bradstreet Reports, July-August, 1980, Volume 28, New York.

4. Pamphlet, Alcohol Abuse and Alcoholism, 1981, National Council on Alcoholism, Delaware Valley Area, Inc.

5. Philadelphia Gay Alcoholics Anonymous Roundup, October 30, 1982.

6. Emma McNally and Dana Finnegan, "Working Together: The National Association of Gay Alcoholism Professionals," *Alcoholism and Homosexuality*, ed. Thomas O. Ziebold. (New York: Haworth Press, 1982), pp. 101–103. NAGAP (The National Association of Gay Alcoholism Professionals) has a directory of facilities and services for gay/lesbian alcoholics and a bibliography. Both are available from NAGAP, 204 W. 20th St., New York, New York 10011.

Homophobic Violence:
Implications for Social Work Practice

Ted R. Bohn

ABSTRACT. Homophobic violence, that is, violence directed at an individual perceived by his/her assailants to be homosexual, is a pervasive social problem in the U.S. Research indicates that anti-gay violence differs markedly from generic violence (that is, violence not motivated by hatred of homosexuals) on several variables. These differences appear to affect the course of treatment and recovery for gay victims, and make necessary specialized interventions. Strategies for service delivery to, and engaging victims of, homophobic violence are considered, as are idiosyncratic clinical concerns, and preventive interventions. The relationship of homophobic violence to the maintenance of the male sex role is also examined.

Although anti-gay violence is an epidemic social problem in the United States, only infrequently have homophobic assaults or homicides received mainstream media attention. Indeed, the phenomenon is carefully concealed from public view for a variety of reasons, not the least of which are the hostility of law enforcement agencies toward homosexual victims, and the lack of concern for homosexual victims evidenced by the media (Bohn, 1982). Only when homophobic violence has reached extremes has the homosexual community responded violently thereby propelling the issue into public consciousness (Hinckle, 1979; Thomas, 1982).

FREQUENCY

Until recently, the indifference or neglect with which the subject was treated by the mainstream media was also evident in scholarly

The author would like to thank Robert Schoenberg and Rick Goldberg for their patience and support in the preparation of this manuscript, as well as the Fund for Human Dignity which supported in part, the research reported herein.

research. The dearth of studies seriously compromised the ability of community organizers to wage effective preventive efforts against homophobic violence, and to establish victims' services for those not fortunate enough to escape it. However, recent research provides some data on the frequency, nature, and scope of anti-gay violence. Bell and Weinberg (1978) for example, found that 38% of white gay men, and 21% of black gay men, in their sample had been robbed or assaulted *at least once*, in connection with their homosexuality.

Harry (1982a) found that 17% of gay men who stated they were "very masculine," 22% of gay men who believed themselves to be "masculine," and 39% of gay men who considered themselves "a little or very feminine," had been violently assaulted by non-gay men. Of those respondents living in gay neighborhoods, furthermore, 27% said they had been assaulted by non-gays, while the figure for gay men living in areas not explicitly identified as gay was 20%. When Harry analyzed the sample on the dimension of "sexual orientation of the victim's friends," he found that 28% of those gay men who stated that all or most of their friends were gay had been beaten by non-gays, while 20% of those who stated that half, most, or all of their friends were straight, had been violently attacked. Harry (1982b) also analyzed victimization on the dimension of childhood and adult cross-gendering, and identified patterns of response similar to those in the previous study.

These findings indicate that anti-gay violence is fairly widespread, affecting 20-40% of the gay male population. The data also suggest that gay males are identifiable to non-gays in a number of ways, including residence in a gay neighborhood, having gay male friends, and non-conformity with traditionally defined male sex role behaviors.

QUALITATIVE DIFFERENCES

Apart from the data on frequency, however, differences in the *nature* of homophobic and generic violence are also telling. Miller and Humphreys (1980) in this regard, reported interesting results in a study of gay male homicide victims. They found that: "In all homicides in the United States during 1976, a knife was employed as the murder weapon in only 17.8% of the cases. Our sample of homosexual victims reveals stabbing as the chief cause of death in

54% of the murders. Only 19% were shot, usually in conjunction with beating or stabbing, another 19% were beaten to death, 6% strangled or smothered, and one was thrown to his death from a roof" (p. 180).

Similarly, Bohn (1983) found that homophobic violence differed on several critical variables from generic violence. For example, whereas most generic assault cases occur between victims and assailants known to each other prior to the incident, slightly more than 93% of homosexual victims of assault or harassment reported that they did not know the perpetrator prior to the incident.

Another difference between generic and homophobic violence is the manner in which the outcome of the incident is guaranteed by the perpetrators *a priori*; that is, the perpetrators seek to insure the defeat/humiliation of their homosexual victims. In the same study, Bohn found that 37% of the assailants of gay men were armed; in another 25% of the cases, the victims were outnumbered by their assailants, and an additional 35% of the cases involved circumstances in which the perpetrators were both armed *and* outnumbered their gay male victims. In only 3% of the reported cases were victims and perpetrators present in equal number, and unarmed.

An analysis of number of perpetrators revealed a mean ratio of 4:1 (perpetrators to homosexual male victims), with a lower limit at 2:1, and an upper limit at 9:1.

While comparative data are unavailable for these measures, this finding strongly suggests that the underlying motive of homophobic assault is to demonstrate heterosexual male superiority vis-à-vis the humiliation and defeat of male homosexuals. The odds for a successful outcome on the homosexual victim's part are virtually eliminated by outnumbering, arming, or both. *Thus do the overwhelming majority of homophobic incidents assume an element of pre-meditation.*

Interestingly, civilian harassment/violence represented only 78% of the reports in this study, with police harassment/brutality accounting for the remaining 22% of reported incidents.

Another hypothesis suggested that victims might be assaulted differentially based on their visibility (a variable conceptually defined on the basis of the victim's associations with other men at the time of the incident). Data showed that 43% of gay males who were assaulted/harassed were alone, 29% were accompanied by one other male, 23.5% were accompanied by more than one male, while only 3% were accompanied by one female, and 1.5% by more than one female. It is evident therefore that gay males were presumed homosexual on the basis of their associations with other men, a finding which was also suggested by Harry's (1982a) research in which sexual orientation of the victim's friends appeared to figure in the likelihood of assault.

MALE RAPE

Rape, whether waged against females or males, is a violent or aggressive act before it is a sexual one, hence its appearance in the realm of homophobic violence. However, unlike heterosexual rape, our society denies that male rape exists, except to the extent that homosexual men are portrayed as rapists of heterosexual men and boys. This notion is not only patently false, but is completely inverted (Scacco, 1982). The overwhelming number of male rapes (note "male" rapes as opposed to "homosexual" rapes), are committed by heterosexual men against gay men or gay youth. The reason for this is that many heterosexual men view male homosexuality as the ultimate form of humiliation; thus, to sexually aggress against a gay man is the ultimate form of negating his masculinity. As with heterosexual rape, the intent is first to overpower and do violence to the victim. This motivational framework attests to the value of homophobic violence in the maintenance of the male sex role.

Researchers also speculate that incidents of male rape are grossly underreported, hence, no reliable measure of its frequency exists. Moreover, a gay male victim of rape rarely comes forward for several reasons: 1) The stigma associated with male rape is formidable and distressing in itself; 2) he may believe that he is the only man who has ever been raped, so imbued with societal denial may he be; 3) he is probably aware (as are most victims of homophobic violence in general) that the police will be apt to respond with hostility if they know he is gay—like the classic oppression of female rape victims, the police will often believe that he wanted to be raped, since he is, after all, a homosexual; 4) he may feel ashamed if he believes (erroneously in most cases) that his assailant(s) were other gay men, or he may be unable to reconcile the notion that other gay men raped him. Most often, however, it will be the case that heterosexual men were responsible for the rape; this is especially true if more than one rapist was involved.

MEN, WOMEN, AND HOMOPHOBIC VIOLENCE

While violence against lesbians does occur, it apparently is not nearly as common as homophobic harassment and assault of male homosexuals. Bell and Weinberg's (1978) data indicated that only 2-5% of homosexual females reported having been assaulted or robbed because of their sexual orientation. Miller and Humphreys (1980) apparently found no cases of female homicide victims. Bohn (1982), with 92% gay male and 8% lesbian victims, replicated the findings of Smith (1981), whose ratio of reported homophobic incidents was 95% male to 5% female. While several researchers have scrutinized their methodologies for possible sampling biases or cultural biases which might tend to skew the data in favor of male respondents, it is believed that the dramatic gender differentials are genuine, and not the result of methodological flaws.

Where sampling strategy involved the use of self-selected samples, advertisements were sent to rape crisis centers and women's organizations in an effort to vigorously encourage lesbian victims to report incidents of homophobic harassment/violence. Those studies utilizing content analyses of homosexual news media, relied heavily upon feminist, women's, and lesbian publications for content, and found even more dramatic gender differentials than availability, readership, or membership samples.

This is not meant to suggest that harassment of, and violence against, lesbians does not occur. However, almost all of the 8% of reports filed by lesbians in the study conducted by Bohn, indicate that harassment and violence against lesbians, occurs in the form of sexual harassment/violence by heterosexual men. Rape is not uncommon, with heterosexual men all the more determined to force their intentions because they view the lesbian as a "challenge" (Norman, 1981). The origins of rape as anti-lesbian violence no doubt derive largely from heterosexual pornography, in which lesbian sexuality is often depicted as prelude to the introduction of a heterosexual male, who eventually conquers both women.

Instrument bias undoubtedly accounts for some of the underrepresentation of lesbians in the results. For example, had researchers framed their questions so as to measure the frequency with which lesbians had been *sexually harassed,* rather than beaten or robbed, the responses would likely have indicated widespread victimization.[1]

These considerations notwithstanding, it is evident that possible methodological flaws can hardly account for gender differentials of this magnitude. Homophobic violence is almost entirely an anti-gay male phenomenon. Indeed, in several instances where lesbians have been violently assaulted, it is because they have been mistaken by their assailants for male homosexuals.[2] In other incidents involving threats and verbal harassment, lesbians have been referred to as "female faggots,"[3] indicating that the incident is justified only to the extent that a resemblance can be found between lesbians and male homosexuals, the latter representing the preferred targets of would-be victimizers. The *meaning* and significance of these dramatic gender differences should not escape analysis. Indeed, the differences suggest a primary function of homophobic violence: enforcement of male sex role norms.

FUNCTIONS OF HOMOPHOBIC VIOLENCE: SCAPEGOATING AND MAINTENANCE OF THE MALE SEX ROLE

The differences between homophobic and generic violence suggest two distinct but not unrelated functions of homophobic violence. The first is simple scapegoating of homosexual males by non-gay males. Allport (1958) describes the process of scapegoating, and the likelihood of violence in situations where scapegoating is treated with impunity by the legal system, and with a considerable degree of social approval. On this view, the objective of homophobic violence is to humiliate, maim, injure, or murder a homosexual individual because of intergroup conflict, resentment, and projection and displacement of anger. This view would find confirmation in several of the differences cited above [e.g., high incidence of police harassment/brutality; the high frequency of arming/outnumbering; and the equally high frequency with which gay victims report that they do not know their assailants prior to the incident, indicating that violence is being perpetrated on one group (gay men) by another group (non-gay men)].

However, a second and equally salient motivation for homophobic assault or harassment can be located in the function of homophobic violence as a primary means of social control, especially as it relates to enforcement of the male sex role. This explanation is supported by differences such as male rape, the *intensity* of the assaults and homicides, dramatic gender differentials, and the vulnerability of victims based on "effeminacy" as well as their associations with other males in public.

This function perhaps weighs most heavily of the two, since if scapegoating were the dominant motivation, we would expect an equal distribution of incidents across the dimension of gender. Moreover, whereas the term "lesbian" is most often thought of as an adjective that describes a certain kind of woman, or actually modifies the word "woman," the terms "gay" and "male" are thought of as antithetical. That is, the male homosexual is portrayed as the *antithesis* of masculinity. At the same time, masculinity is an attribute which can never be proved once-and-for-all, but in fact, must be proved over and over again everyday. Thus, for those bent on *machismo*, one way of proving masculinity is to destroy its antithesis, namely, the male homosexual, which ipso facto confers masculine status by default.

As a result of these considerations, the remainder of this article will be confined to male homosexual victims. It shall be the thesis of this article that the qualitative differences that distinguish homophobic violence from generic violence, can not help but impact upon the male homosexual, and that homophobic violence demands a distinct response from social work practitioners. Community organizing strategies, casework functions, and groupwork activities are examined. Also considered are clinical issues peculiar to homophobic victimization.

SOCIAL WORK METHOD

The three traditional methods of social work intervention, community organization, casework, and groupwork, each have their place in social work with victims of homophobic violence.

Community Organizing and Prevention

In the context of homophobic violence, community organizing is equivalent to prevention. Community organizing against homophobic violence takes place through the establishment of local violence projects [e.g., the New York City Gay/Lesbian Anti-Violence Project (formerly the Chelsea Gay Association), and San Francisco's Community United Against Violence (CUAV), among others]. These projects maintain offices and 24 hour hotlines in their respective municipalities and provide an array of victim's services which are considered below.

The purposes of the local projects are two-fold. The first is the collection of data on anti-gay violence. Because homophobic violence is ignored as a social problem, and (research oriented) funding agencies have committed little money to funding studies of homophobic violence, little data and research are presently available. Law enforcement agencies in most localities, out of institutional homophobia, deny that homophobic violence exists. In some cases, police departments classify homophobic crimes as "assaults or homicides without motive," although they know that heterosexual-homosexual antagonisms account for the incident. Other institutions too deny the existence of homophobic violence (e.g., the courts, district attorneys, etc.). Consequently, data-collection is an extremely important function of local violence projects. The second purpose of these projects is to provide victim's services.

The data collected by local violence projects can assist gay activists and community-organizers in documenting program proposals for victim's services as well as providing the basis for arguments in favor of gay rights legislation. It is because of the critical role that data of this variety ultimately play in prevention, that every victim of homophobic violence should be encouraged to report the incident to the local project, and then to the police, Internal Affairs Division, or Civilian Complaint Review Board.

Local projects also target the society as the population in need of intervention, and strategize accordingly. One strategy for the prevention of homophobic violence is to organize gay street patrols. For example, San Francisco has organized two such patrols, which function not as vigilante groups, but as organized units of gay men and lesbians who patrol the streets with walkie-talkies. They are frequently able to avert homophobic incidents by ushering the perpetrator(s) to the border of the gay neighborhood, or by contacting police. The patrols have proved extremely successful.

Another community organizing strategy is to organize self-defense classes for gay men and lesbians. Such classes presently exist in several U.S. cities, and are offered free of cost or at reduced rates. Self-defense classes are an important way of overcoming helplessness, as well as gaining confidence. While an ability to defend onself may not obviate homophobic violence, it nonetheless can prevent an incident from continuing.

Violence projects also provide liaison to the local police department. If the police in a community are uncooperative or hostile, then local violence projects often assume the role of advocate, and organize demonstrations against the police, or work with the city administration to force the police to be more responsive to the gay community. If the police are cooperative, then liaisons are generally established between the police and the project. The project may assist the police in solving crimes and homicides, and providing training sessions which sensitize new police recruits to gay/lesbian issues.

Violence projects also provide the very necessary service of court-monitoring.[4] Few gay victims ever report homophobic violence to the police (fearing secondary reprisals or recriminations from the police themselves). Thus, the projects also laboriously attempt to convince victims to file complaints with the police.

However, local projects soon discovered that after investing considerable energy in persuading a victim to file charges, that the district attorney would fail to prosecute for "lack of motive" (which really meant "lack of concern for a homosexual male victim"); if the case managed to get to court, it would often be prosecuted with extreme leniency, or dismissed by equally homophobic judges.[5] An effective strategy is to monitor the court calendar and to fill the courtroom with gay male and lesbian onlookers. Of equal importance is the practice of providing information on homophobic violence to judges (who may otherwise impose an unusually light sentence). This strategy too has proved extremely efficacious and resulted in sentences that are more severe.

Local projects will also attempt to promote prevention on the legislative level. Data from violence projects have been used to argue for gay rights legislation in several U.S. cities, on the premise that any policy that protects the rights of gay men and lesbians will diminish homophobic violence. Two other types of legislative goals also exist. The first is legislation which establishes criminal penalties for homophobic or sexual assault or slurs. Such legislation already protects individuals from racial and ethnic slurs/assault in at least one county in the U.S., and its enforcement has been occasioned by community endorsement.[6] Local projects have increasingly come to recognize the need for legislation which bans sexual slurs or assaults with criminal liability. A second legislative initiative is to introduce legislation which authorizes homosexual victims to file civil suits against their assailants. While many states already authorize civil actions for racist, sexist, or other forms of assault, the only known bill which extends such privilege to homosexual victims is presently pending before the California state legislature.[7]

Finally, and perhaps most important of all primary prevention efforts, is public education. Schools have also been the targets of educational efforts aimed at demystifying the homosexual, since it is in the secondary schools largely that cultural norms and mores related to sex role structure and homosexuality are transmitted. Public media are also enlisted in an effort to force the issue of homophobic violence into public consciousness. Part of the problem is that non-gays are unaware of the frequency and severity of the phenomenon, and fail to assist in its prevention.

CASEWORK

Workers in local projects often function as caseworkers with many and varied functions. If the victim requires medical attention, for example, the worker will assist him in negotiating the medical/insurance bureaucracies. If the victim has no insurance, the worker will assist him in making application to state victim's agencies which, as the payor of last resort, will usually assume the cost of medical bills, provided the victim can show that the injuries were the result of a violent assault or robbery. In the event of homicide, the worker can assist a lover or other survivors in making funeral arrangements, and in filing for compensation from state victim's agencies which may assume funeral costs if the victim died as a result of injuries sustained in a violent assault.

Essentially, the philosophy of local anti-gay violence projects is that no victim of homophobic violence should ever have to bear the costs associated with recovery, since anti-gay violence is a *social* (and hence societal) problem. A gay victim should hardly be expected to bear the monetary costs of societal homophobia in addition to the physical and emotional toll of an assault.

If the victim has been followed by his assailants to his home, or, if the incident took place in the victim's home, the worker may also stay with him until such time as he is able to locate alternative quarters. At that time, the worker may assist the victim in moving to another apartment.

Since the victim is referred to the worker through the violence hotline, the victim can usually be expected to be in a state of crisis. After the initial crisis has been diminished somewhat, and the worker has made the victim feel safe, it will also be the worker's function to attempt to convince the victim to file charges/complaint with the appropriate agency: the police in the case of civilian violence/harassment, and either the Police Internal Affairs Division or the Civilian Complaint Review Board in the case of police harassment/brutality. This may be entirely impracticable for some victims whose family relations, jobs, or other essential systems could not withstand the effects of publicity. However, the possibility of filing charges/complaints should always be explored.

For victims who are "out," the prospect of publicity should not be an obstacle to filing charges/complaints. Indeed, if the individual agrees, the worker may want to seek coverage of the incident in the mainstream media, so that the case also serves the function of public education. These decisions, however, can only be made by the victim, although they deserve the help of the worker.

If the individual agrees to file a complaint/charge, he may require the worker's assistance, since he is already in a state of heightened vulnerability as a result of the crisis, and because the police are frequently uncooperative if not hostile to victims of homophobic assault. The worker will therefore serve as a mediator and advocate for the victim in filing a complaint.

The caseworker will also be responsible for subsequent monitoring of the case with the D.A.'s office, as well as the courts and the detectives assigned to the case, since cases involving homosexual victims are famous for "disappearing" or remaining inactive for protracted periods of time, until finally dismissed. If it appears that the case is being "stalled," or ignored, this should be openly discussed in case meetings, and pressure brought to bear on the police/D.A.

The caseworker should also assess the presence or absence of a support network. If the victim's lover or friends can support him in some tasks (e.g., staying with him, helping him move, etc.), they should then be enlisted. In the absence of any support systems, the caseworker must assume friendship/kinship roles as well.

The worker can also facilitate entry into ancillary services such as self-defense classes and counseling. Counseling is an integral part of recovery for many victims and may take the form of individual, family, couple, or group work. Although concrete services should receive immediate attention from the worker, the clinical issues involved in recovery are equally important.

CLINICAL CONSIDERATIONS

Most victims of homophobic assault report that they would utilize counseling services if they were available.[8] While other services are essential and may take priority over counseling, it is important to realize that assault can produce many feelings and thoughts which are difficult to accept.

The Aftermath

It is precisely because homophobic violence differs from generic violence in its intensity that a survivor may well experience the aftermath with greater intensity than the victim of generic violence. Miller and Humphreys (1980) state: "That intense rage is present in nearly all homicide cases with homosexual victims is evident. A striking feature of most murders in this sample is their gruesome, often vicious nature. Seldom is a homosexual victim simply shot. He is more apt to be stabbed a dozen times, mutilated, *and* strangled" (p. 179).

This intensity of rage also characterizes non-homicidal homophobic incidents. Homophobic rage produces in the survivor, equally intense reactions. A gay male victim can generally be expected to exhibit many of the same symptoms seen in female rape victims: feeling as though he is "bad" or inadequate, that he somehow deserved or invited the attack, or that he is in some other way responsible. Many victims feel intense guilt, embarrassment, shame, depression, and also experience a complete loss of confidence. He may also experience feelings of terror following a violent attack, as well as paranoia (manifest in locking all doors and windows and getting up during the night to check them several times), or a refusal to leave the home. These feelings and behaviors can persist for several months or years if they are not acknowledged and worked through.

Negative feelings of this sort do not always appear within hours or days of an incident. There may be a substantial delay of weeks or even months between the incident and the emergence of these feelings.

The worker should also be acutely aware of signs of suicidal ideation or attempts. Homophobic assault can leave a victim feeling as though there is absolutely no reason to continue living. This appears to be especially true in instances where the victim is not "out of the closet." Miller and Humphreys again provide insight on this score:

> Being victimized is often cause for guilt, but being victimized in the course of pursuing socially devalued goals produces concomitantly greater guilt and shame. Many homosexual father respondents seriously confronted their homosexuality for the first time as a result of suffering criminal victimization. In being attacked, they did not so much come out of the closet as have the closet involuntarily ripped from around them. Such unanticipated exposure may be psychologically devastating. Two homosexual fathers, for instance, report having considered suicide after such experiences." (p. 178)

This view is reiterated by Rofes (1983) who demonstrates the ways in which victimization may lead ultimately to suicide, and who provides several case examples.

Major depressions are also not unusual, and it may require time for any desire to live to return. Loss of motivation and other depressive symptomatology can frequently be observed. A significant amount of depressive feelings stem from the often ardent denial that follows an incident. If the victim is extremely depressed, he has probably still not *accepted* (unconditionally) the incident. Thus, a major objective of counseling victims of homophobic assault is to help the victim accept the fact that he was victimized (note: this is not an argument for helping the victim to accept *homophobia;* instead, it is the reality of the *incident* that must be accepted). As long as the victim consciously or unconsciously resists acknowledging the incident or its emotional legacy, the work of the aftermath awaits him.

Empathy and compassion are also important aspects of counseling victims of homophobic violence. The victim needs to be comforted and made to feel safe. He will need to experience the uncomfortable feelings which will almost invariably accompany acceptance. The therapist should not avoid experiencing these feelings along with the victim, and should closely examine any resistance s/he has to sharing the experience with a victim.

However, by no means should the client's state of heightened vulnerability be entirely accepted. While a certain amount of withdrawal and isolation are to be expected, efforts should also be made to give the victim emotional support and contact. This may represent a particularly dangerous problem for the gay male victim, who, disgusted with the costs of being gay, withdraws from other gay people following a violent homophobic incident. The therapist should in fact encourage the victim to utilize or create an extended gay support network rather than withdrawing from other gay people. This support network will survive and emerge as a functional system long after the crisis of homophobic assault is lessened. It can and should develop without conditions of obligation or indebtedness.

Furthermore, gay male victims of rape need to be helped to understand the dynamics of male rape. Client education is thus an important aspect of recovery. Because our society ignores male rape or perpetuates the notion that homosexual men rape other men, the gay male victim may well hold the very same beliefs about male rape as are socially prominent. Such a belief system can adversely affect a gay male victim's image of self and of other gay men, and seriously complicate recovery (e.g., by way of alcoholism, etc.). These may have a negative impact on his interactions with other gay men. He must therefore be made aware of what rape means to heterosexual male rapists, and why it is likely that the rapist was not gay.

Groupwork

Social workers use a variety of methods in working with victims of homophobic violence, including casework, individual and couple counseling, and community organization. All are effective ways of helping victims of homophobic violence to work through the feelings described earlier and to meet the victim's concrete needs. However, another method that appears to be even more successful in this regard, is groupwork. It is this method that permits the victim not simply the opportunity to explore and work through the feelings he has about himself, other gay people, the assailants, and the incident itself, but allows him to engage in the essential process of *identification* with other victims. In this way, victims can express their anger, share their reactions with other victims, and know that they are not alone in the work of recovery. Although individual or couple counseling can help victims to experience their feelings of disgust, inadequacy, responsibility, anger, and fear, group experiences have the added benefit of support from other victims, which individual and couple counseling do not always provide.

Yet another method, perhaps most successful of all, is to combine group work with individual counseling, so that in addition to identifying with other victims in a group setting, the individual has a private session in which he can explore feelings that were not able to be considered in group, either because of time constraints or because the individual felt too threatened to confront them in the presence of other victims. Group experiences can occasionally become too "dilute," in which case victims should also feel free to seek individual sessions which focus solely on him.

The outcomes or objectives of counseling should include helping the victim regain his self-confidence, coming to see himself as a survivor rather than as a victim, and restoring feelings of competence and wholeness, while diminishing feelings of guilt, shame, helplessness, and embarrassment.

Discharge of anger is also an important function of counseling, since a victim may experience delayed anger or rage at his assailants. If not appropriately acknowledged, anger may be directed at other gay people, including friends and lovers, or internalized and directed at oneself.

Attributional Styles

Although most violent incidents appear to create in the victim some need to assess blame/responsibility for the incident, the case of homophobic violence is especially problematic. For the historical stigma associated with male homosexuality has left an unconscious residue of guilt in many gay male victims;[9] this residue is often elicited by homophobic incidents. The attributions which gay men use to explain a homophobic attack are susceptible to manipulation by residual feelings of guilt.

A victim may exhibit several attributional styles in assessing responsibility for the incident. Four are defined here. These are: unconscious-internal (where the victim has blamed himself for the incident without knowing it); unconscious-external (the victim has blamed someone else, either the assailants, a friend or lover, for the incident without knowing it); conscious-internal (the victim has blamed himself for the incident and has done so knowingly); and conscious-external (the blame is assessed against someone else, knowingly). The unconscious attributions will now be examined/illustrated with case examples.

Case I. Peter, a 19 year old gay male who was beaten by a group of 4 heterosexual men in their mid-20s, presents to a local violence project for counseling related to the incident. His statements about the assault reveal that on some level, he believes that he was "too visible" as a male homosexual. The focus of his statements concern his mannerisms, which he considers "effeminate." When asked whether he believes he deserved the assault, he quickly and somewhat angrily answers that he does not. Yet he consistently indicates that his mannerisms make him identifiably gay, and that if these could be changed, he wouldn't be quite so vulnerable.

The client's attributional style then is unconscious-internal, and he needs to be helped to explore the reasons for self-blame. A treatment dilemma exists here as well. On the one hand, it is true that males who exhibit "effeminate" traits are significantly more likely to be the victims of homophobic violence than males who do not (Harry, 1982a). Thus, his behaviors place him at "high-risk" for assault by non-gay men. However, these facts attest to the social-control functions of homophobic violence, and demonstrate that anti-gay violence serves to enforce rigid definitions of "appropriate" (i.e., heterosexually-defined) male sex role behavior. What is essential in spite of the dilemma, however, is that the unconscious self-blame be brought into consciousness, so that the youth can next absolve himself of guilt or responsibility for the incident, and thereafter decide how to minimize future risk. Perhaps rather than discouraging, punishing, or eliminating "feminine" behaviors from his repertoire, thus fulfilling the intent of the violenct act, the client could be enrolled in ongoing self-defense classes, so that he could retain "feminine" behaviors, and still minimize risk.

Case II. A gay couple (Jim and Steve) are assaulted after leaving their apartment in a gay neighborhood. Both members of the couple were hospitalized for a week, with several broken bones and a concussion between them. They are referred from the social work services department of the hospital to a local violence project, and from there to a gay counseling agency which has agreed to accept such cases free of charge on referral from the violence project. It soon becomes apparent to the worker that one partner (Jim) has an unconscious belief about the incident: "We were only identifiable as gay because we were walking together." In this way, the other partner (Steve) is covertly blamed for the incident, since without him, the assailants might not have identified them as a homosexual couple, and the incident might never have happened.

The attributional style is unconscious-external. While Jim will reduce his own sense of guilt by way of this attribution, he will create enduring problems in the relationship without knowing it. The couple needs to receive counseling from a worker who can help them resolve the incident without placing blame on each other. Again, the unconscious attribution (one of blame projected onto the other partner), must be explored and brought into consciousness. Its possible recurrence must be anticipated in future interactions since it is likely that this attributional style will persist for some time. The couple also needs to be educated and convinced that they have the right to walk together as a couple. Only the values and judgments placed on their relationship by non-gay others are in need of change, not their desire to be together.

Other problems may emerge if the incident involved a couple. For example, one of the primary manifestations of homophobia is the disdain its proponents hold for intimacy of any kind between males. Consequently, homophobic violence can have the effect of interfering with a couple's intimacy. If either or both are unconsciously or consciously blaming the other for the incident, intimacy will inevitably suffer. Counseling may therefore involve intimacy issues as well.

If either or both individuals blame *himself* for the incident, the effect may be one of complete withdrawal. On the other hand, an equally frequent manifestation of homophobic violence is "clinging" behavior, in which one or both partners becomes overly dependent upon the other. The behavior is so exaggerated that the couple may withdraw as a "unit," from all social contact; these dependencies may be heavily resistant to exploration. Thus, in one instance a violent homophobic incident may have the effect of interfering with male-male intimacy, and in another, may have the paradoxical effect of creating mutually-exclusive dependencies that are not likely to be amenable to rapid change.

A final complication may result if one partner reacts with "clinging" behavior, and the other reacts by withdrawing. It is usually the case in this configuration that partner #1 has blamed himself for the incident, while partner #2 has blamed partner #1. The differences in attributional style may or may not reflect similar differences in the relationship.

Attributing responsibility for a homophobic incident to a friend or partner is simply projecting social responsibility onto another individual because the victim has a need to blame someone, perhaps even that specific person. If a victim blames himself, he is simply retroflecting the blame rather than making an appropriate attribution to the individual assailants and the environment that encourages homophobic assault. Blame then becomes a central issue in the aftermath of a homophobic incident. And because of the residue of guilt that lies waiting in gay men, internal attributions need to be expunged. With few exceptions attributions should be geared toward conscious-external targets (i.e., the assailants).

Furthermore, gay men who are comfortable with their sexuality have most often arrived at this relative peace through a protracted process of acceptance (Berger, 1983), during which a lifetime of negative societal messages are rejected in favor of a homosexual identity. This process of early acceptance in gay men has been viewed as a positive dynamic in later life transitions and challenges (e.g., in aging). However, the victim who blames himself for a homophobic incident may also come to *accept* self-blame or victim-status as a result of previous internal acceptance processes. The worker should be careful that victims do not simply accept self-blame, but instead, accept only the incident.

Thus, counseling victims of homophobic violence is both directive and non-directive. The client should not be directed until he begins to make inappropriate attributions, or, in the judgment of the worker, requires client education about homosexuality or the nature of homophobia.

Two components of the attribution then need to be assessed: the locus of control (internal-external) and whether the attribution is conscious or unconscious. Most often, attributions in these cases will be unconscious. It becomes the worker's task to help the victim bring the attribution into consciousness, and next examine the need to blame oneself. It is generally not until the victim understands that the assailants and the social environment are responsible for the incident that he begins to feel anger. (Interestingly, violence workers report that many gay victims experience a latency of weeks or months before reporting an incident to a gay hotline or violence project. This latency is now thought to correspond to the emergence of anger in the victim. At the same time, anger accompanies the abandonment of denial.)

The Male and Homosexual Interface

Although many gay men have rejected harmful stereotypes of masculinity, other pernicious behaviors survive unnoticed. For example, American society socializes males to believe that they should be strong enough to defend themselves. Indeed, the ability to defend oneself is an inherent measure of a man's self-worth (David and Brannon, 1976; Lewis, 1978; Petras, 1975). Not surprisingly then, the gay male victim of violence will often experience feelings of guilt, inadequacy, shame, or self-hatred following physical assault, for he has probably come to view his victimization as an indication of failure or weakness. The attribution is almost immediately recognizable as internal and unconscious, and the consequences can be devastating. (The assumption is that he could not triumph because of the outnumbering/arming antics of homophobic perpetrators).

However, in addition to the message that says "I should have been strong enough to defend myself," other harmful sex-role messages often contaminate recovery. Because men are taught that they must be ever strong, a gay male victim will probably also believe that he should be able to help himself afterwards. Thus, in addition to blaming himself for not having defended himself "adequately," he may also expect to be able to handle self-blame and similar feelings afterwards. Patterns such as this ("I can handle my own problems/I should be able to handle my own problems") resemble many of the difficulties males in therapy may have (Goldberg, 1976). So pervasive is the injunction against seeking help for males, that often following an attack, a gay man will simply find himself *unable* to ask for help (especially from other gay men, whom he may believe also view his victimization as weakness).

Because of sex role pressure which insists that vulnerability never be exposed in front of other men, a victim may in fact conceal an assault from other gay men, friends, or lovers, and carry the self-blame and humiliation around in silence. He may avoid asking for help from a hotline, counselor, or violence project. If such cases are known, it is appropriate for the social worker to contact the victim and offer counseling or other victim's services. Proferring services as a method (Germain and Gitterman, 1980), however, may be inherently problematic in the case of homophobic violence. Extreme caution must be used if the intervention is offered, for inviting a victim to utilize counseling or other services may be viewed by the victim as an implicit statement of his weakness, and have the effect of increasing guilt.

Whether the victim seeks help will depend most intricately upon his reaction to the assault. If he reacts in the not uncommon way of withdrawing completely, then services can and should be proferred. The majority of males only seek help in periods of intolerable crisis, that is, they do not seek preventive help, but wait until the problem becomes disruptive or unmanageable in their own lives. Most often such clients will only remain in therapy long enough to realize some symptom alleviation, and then terminate abruptly. Gay male clients who are in crisis, or who have internalized messages which imply that men should be able to handle their own problems, probably have a difficult time viewing themselves as worthy of help, and need to be reassured that asking for help is entirely natural.

Thus, in addition to the ego-disruptions that crisis or trauma may cause, the incident may precipitate further identity crises by requiring of the victim violations of proscribed male sex role behaviors (i.e., allowing oneself to be dependent upon another individual, exposing one's vulnerability, etc.).

Finally, a gay male victim may, because of socialization aimed at making him totally self-sufficient, enter into a prolonged period of emotional denial following an assault. Denying the distress caused by the incident, however, only defers confronting the pain and humiliation which do not dissipate of their own accord. The emotions, although difficult to acknowledge, need to be explored, experienced, and finally accepted. Recovery is nearly complete when the victim has accepted the incident as well as the attendant feelings it produced, but has disowned the pattern of victim-thinking that has made him afraid of life.

CONCLUSION

Anti-gay violence is an epidemic social problem in the U.S. It has created considerable need in the gay community, and demands a distinct response from social workers. Victims of homophobic violence can however be helped to recover from assault-trauma through individual counseling or groupwork. However, the need for funding of local violence projects which document such incidents and provide victim's services is acute. Social workers can become involved in prevention at the primary, secondary, and tertiary levels, and include in legislative lobbying efforts, the need for legislation which specifically addresses homophobic violence and which establishes both criminal and civil liability for the perpetrators.

NOTES

1. Such a study is presently underway at the National Gay Task Force Violence Project.

2. An article in *Gay Community News* (Boston), describes the beating of two lesbians, whose assailants mistook them for a gay male couple. Anti-gay male epithets were used during the incident, despite the attempts of the women to expose the error.

3. The November, 1981 issue of *Womanews* contains a hate letter sent to the proprietors of the Lesbian Herstory Archives in New York. The letter begins: "To the two female faggots, I hate fags of both sexes, and my campaign of terror against you has only just begun."

4. The practice of court-monitoring was first devised and introduced by the Chelsea Gay Association's Anti-Violence Project (NYC).

5. A case involving a gay man named Richard Heakin in the late 1970s serves as a paradigm example of judicial homophobia. Heakin was standing outside of a gay bar in Tucson, when a carload of four heterosexual men drove up. Its occupants got out and beat Heakin to death. Although the four freely admitted to having murdered Heakin because he was gay, the judged dismissed the charges against them, calling them "model athletes."

6. Nassau County, N.Y.

7. Assembly Bill number 848.

8. Conclusion of training sessions for the National Gay Task Force Violence Project. The Project conducts an ongoing national study of anti-gay violence, and has a toll-free telephone number for this purpose.

9. The author is indebted to Michael Lynch for this observation. Lynch addressed guilt in the context of Kaposi's Sarcoma and A.I.D.S., in an article titled "Living with Kaposi's" in the November, 1982 issue of *The Body Politic*.

REFERENCES

Allport, G. *The nature of prejudice*. New York: Doubleday Anchor Books, 1958.

Bell, A.P. and Weinberg, M.S. *Homosexualities: A study of diversity among men and women*. New York: Simon and Schuster, 1978.

Berger, R.M. What is a homosexual?: A definitional model. *Social Work,* 1983, Vol. 28, No. 2, 132-135.

Bohn, T.R. Violence against gay men and lesbians: America's best kept secret. *The Connection,* 1982, Vol. 2, No. 6.

Bohn, T.R. Violence against gay men and lesbians: Empirical research on trends in homophobic violence. (Unpublished Master's thesis, School of Social Welfare, State University of New York at Stony Brook), 1983.

David, D.S. and Bronnon, R. (Eds.) *The forty-nine percent majority: The male sex role*. Reading, Ma.: Addison-Wesley Publishing Company, 1976.

Germain, C.B. and Gitterman, A. *The life model of social work practice*. New York: Columbia University Press, 1980.

Goldberg, H. *The hazards of being male: Surviving the myth of masculine privilege*. New York: Signet, 1976.

Harry, J. Derivative deviance: The cases of extortion, fag-bashing, and shakedown of gay men. *Criminology,* February, 1982a, Vol. 19, No. 4, pp. 546-564.

Harry, J. *Gay children grown up: Gender culture and gender deviance*. New York: Praeger Publishers, 1982b.

Hinckle, W. Dan White's San Francisco: The untold story. *Inquiry,* October 29, 1979.

Lewis, R.A. Emotional intimacy among men. *Journal of Social Issues,* 1978, Vol. 34, No. 1, pp. 108-121.

Miller, B. and Humphreys, L. Lifestyles and violence: Homosexual victims of assault and murder. *Qualitative Sociology,* Fall, 1980, Vol. 3, No. 3, pp. 169-185.

Norman, A. The problem of violence. *Catalyst,* Winter, 1981, Vol. 3, No. 4, pp. 83-90.

Petras, J.M. *Sex male, gender masculine: Selected readings in male sexuality*. New York: Alfred Publishing Co., 1975.

Rofes, E. *Lesbians, gay men and suicide*. San Francisco: Grey Fox Press, 1983.

Scacco, A.M., Jr. (Ed.) *Male rape: A casebook of sexual aggressions*. New York: AMS Press, Inc., 1982.

Smith, R.J. Report to the Governor's Task Force on Civil Rights. Presented on behalf of the Community United Against Violence (CUAV), San Francisco, CA., November, 1981.

Thomas, D.J. San Francisco's 1979 White Night Riot: Injustice, vengeance, and beyond. In Paul, W., Weinrich, J.D., Gonsiorek, J.C., and Hotvedt, M.E., (Eds.), *Homosexuality: Social, psychological, and biological issues*. Beverly Hills: Sage Publications, 1982, pp. 337-350.

III

Professional Issues

Homophobia:
A Study of the Attitudes
of Mental Health Professionals
Toward Homosexuality

Teresa A. DeCrescenzo

ABSTRACT. A 20-page questionnaire was administered to 140 mental health professionals employed in a variety of service delivery agencies, both public and private. Respondents were asked a variety of demographic questions covering 23 variables, and were asked their opinions on a number of issues related to attitudes toward homosexuality. Statistically significant differences were found among various disciplines and within disciplines on certain items. The findings illuminate some sources of attitude development, including family of origin, religious background, parental education level and other sources as well. A 9-item "homophobia scale" emerged, which achieved a Guttman Scalogram coefficient of reproducibility of .96.

Using Weinberg's (1972) definition of homophobia, this study was designed to measure the incidence of homophobic attitudes among mental health practitioners, and to correlate the extent to which those attitudes are impacted by such variables as age, sex, education, income, religion, social class and sources of professional and social stimulation.

According to Weinberg, the fear of homosexuality is inculcated early in life, and can be expressed as antagonism toward a particular group of people, as self-loathing in the case of homosexuals themselves, or through the support of repressive laws designed to eliminate homosexual behavior.

Clearly, overt support of legislation which attempts to discriminate against, or restrict the behavior of, homosexuals is readily identifiable. Less easily isolated are the more subtle behaviors and beliefs which are manifestations of incipient homophobia. For example, the therapist who invites a homosexual client, whose present life situation is unsatisfying, to consider the possibility that the genesis of the dissatisfaction may be a function of the client's sexual orientation would not likely be responsive to being labelled "homophobic." Yet, while one frequently hears of the necessity for homosexual clients to reexamine their sexual orientation, one rarely hears of heterosexual clients being asked to reconsider their sexual orientation.

Given the difficulty of empirically demonstrating the existence of homophobia, the few experiments which are reported in the literature are noteworthy. In 1967, McConaghy designed a device to identify male homosexuals through the measurement of penile volume change in response to viewing suggestive pictures of nude men and women. The homosexual males experienced no penile volume change in response to pictures of nude women, and showed marked increase in penile volume when showed pictures of nude men. Similarly, the heterosexual males experienced an increase in penile volume when shown suggestive pictures of nude women, however, these same males suffered a homophobic reaction when shown pictures of nude men, and their penises actually shrank. While it is true that men routinely experience penile volume change even when not in a sexually charged environment, the degree of change on the part of heterosexual males in response to suggestive pictures of nude men suggests that their reaction was one of fear.

Morin (1975) conducted an experiment to determine how near people would want to come to a person whom they believed to be homosexual. Both males and females selected actual physical distances which were significantly greater for where they wanted to be seated in relation to a person whom they suspected was homosexual, than the distances they chose to seat themselves from a presumed heterosexual.

Perhaps the most telling experiment in the area of identifying homophobia was conducted by Karr (1975). He arranged, by collaboration, to have one person disclose in a group setting that someone else was a homosexual (in fact, that person was not). Subjects in the experiment were asked to rate each other on various attributes, and the identified homosexual was rated as being more vain, superficial and effeminate than he was during a separate phase of the experiment in which the same person was not identified as a homosexual. It appears that the label created the perception of deviance. Interestingly, the collaborators who arranged for the false disclosure were rated as being more sociable and more masculine than they had been rated in the phase of the experiment during which they did not identify anyone in terms of sexual orientation. It appears, then, that males are rewarded by others in contemporary society when they denigrate homosexuals.

Speculation on the causes of homophobia have not yielded empirical evidence in this area, though the destructive effects of this phenomenon have been extensively documented (Weinberg, 1972; Berzon and Clark, 1975; Freedman, 1976; Berzon, 1976; Clark, 1977; and others).

SOCIETAL RESPONSES TO HOMOSEXUAL BEHAVIOR

Societal responses to homosexual behavior around the world have been irregular throughout history, and are often found to be coincident with upheaval and major changes in a society. Injunctions against homosexual behavior have undergone numerous metamorphoses, from religious proscriptions, to laws, to psychological theories.

During the time of the Inquisition, which began in Spain and moved across the face of Europe into Belgium and The Netherlands, church courts were held to try infidels. Homosexuals were often found to be infidels, and were sentenced to be burned at the stake. Although the "separation of church and state" doctrine evolved from the abuses of the Inquisition, the actual divorce between church and state was, and still is, a slow process. Laws defining homosexual acts as criminal behavior were frequently written in biblical terms, for example, the State of Virginia still describes sodomy as "an abominable crime against nature," with no further description or explanation of the act.

After Truman's precipitious rise to the presidency, at a time when the psychic atmosphere in America was highly charged with fear, Senator Joseph P. McCarthy introduced a Congressional resolution declaring contemporary art to be subversive. Later, he appeared in Senate chambers with a list, which he stated contained the names of 650 persons working in the State Department who were subversive because they were homosexuals.

While socialists, pacifists and labor union organizers were also among McCarthy's targets, he was particularly vitriolic in his attacks against homosexuals. There has been considerable speculation in the media in recent years that McCarthy might himself have been a homosexual, lending credence to Weinberg's assertion that the self-loathing experienced by some homosexuals causes them to suffer from an attitude of revulsion and anger toward things homosexual. This concept seems to apply to other public figures who invested considerable energy in anti-homosexual activities as well, such as the late FBI Director, J. Edgar Hoover, and Harry Stack Sullivan, American-born psychoanalytic theorist whose private life was tormented by his own homosexual tendencies, according to a recently published biography (1982).

When Hitler began organizing the Lumpen proletariat in the mid-1920s, in the face of mass joblessness, double digit inflation and the lack of leadership from the ageing Von Hindenberg, one class of people whom he took into his cells was homosexual. Ernst Rohm, a key tactician and strategist of the "Brown Shirts," was a known homosexual, who was later slain when the purge of homosexuals began in 1934, during the "Night of the Long Knives" (Lauritsen and Thorstad, 1974). The subsequent detention, trial and execution of nearly 250,000 homosexuals, identified in the concentration camps by wearing a pink triangle on the left shoulder or leg, have been widely documented elsewhere. Many Latin countries, embarrassed by the presence of men who did not appear to carry out the tradition of "machismo," have severely penalized suspected homosexuals. After the socialist revolution in Cuba, homosexuals were denounced as "bourgeoisie decadent," and identified male homosexuals were incarcerated in "reeducation centers." In 1965, large numbers of male homosexuals were forcibly marched through the streets of Havana, wearing signs tied around their necks which read "yo soy un puto" (I am a whore). A document protesting this treatment signed by noted social activists such as Simone de Beauvoir and Jean Genet was delivered to Fidel Castro. As a result, Cuba's extreme position with regard to homosexuals has softened somewhat, but homosexual behavior is still not sanctioned in Cuba.

The circular metamorphosis from religion to law to mental health practice was completed in the United States with the adoption of psychoanalytic theory. From around the turn of the century and during the first one-third of the 20th century, mainly through the work of Charcot, Breuer, Freud and Mesmer, homosexuality was viewed as being neither simple nor criminal, it was simply a sickness.

The "sickness" model officially persisted until the removal of homosexuality from the list of mental disorders in psychiatric nomenclature in 1973. Homosexuality, at that time, was listed as "sexual orientation disturbance," until the recent third edition of the Diagnostic and Statistical Manual (DSM III), which reflects the diagnostic category of "ego-dystonic homosexuality."

During recent years, there has been a surge of new efforts to resume the circular metamorphosis from mental health to sin and back to law with respect to homosexual behavior. For example, in 1978, Dade County, Florida, repealed an ordinance granting equal job and housing protection to homosexuals (the major thrust of the campaign theme was the need to bring "local ordinances into line with God's law"). In 1979, Californians defeated a piece of legislation designed to prohibit homosexuals and those who advocate homosexuality from being hired as teachers in California schools (as in the Dade County campaign, proponents of this legislation used biblical quotes to establish their legal position). In 1980, federal legislators upheld the Immigration and Naturalization Service's decision to refuse entry into the United States to a British gay newspaper reporter who attempted to attend a gay event in San Francisco. The decision affirmed that "Congress clearly intended to prohibit homosexuals from residing in the United States." One factor in this fairly recent decision was the Surgeon General's decision that homosexuality is an illness, and customs officials must not knowingly permit sick people to cross America's borders.

ATTITUDES OF MENTAL HEALTH PRACTITIONERS

Clearly, the attitudes of mental health practitioners have implications, not only for how homosexuals will be treated by such professionals, but also for future legislation in the area of social control. Homophobia is an important research topic and much can be learned through the consideration of the various ingredients which contribute to the attitudes people develop toward homosexual behavior.

It is important to discuss what homophobia is, to discover the extent to which it exists among mental health practitioners and to determine the impact it may have on the degree of social and legal pressures brought to bear on homosexuals. Though homophobia can take many forms, ranging from the pogroms of Hitler and the Inquisition, to the quiet desperation of a furtive sexual contact in a public restroom, the main foci of this study are the existence of homophobia among mental health professionals, the implications of therapist attitude on the quality of client-therapist interaction and possible ways to counteract the effects of homophobia.

Clearly, attitudes and values affect the ways in which humans interact, and that axiom extends to the interaction between client and therapist as well. Most mental health professionals would agree that there is no such thing as "value-free" therapy. In fact, from an historical perspective, one might observe that psychoanalysis has been, in part, a social control agent, reflecting prevailing social mores, helping the deviant to become more socially acceptable both in behavior and in attitude.

If, then, it should be demonstrated that a significant degree of homophobia exists among some mental health professionals, there will be concern regarding behaviors toward homosexual clients. The probability is that homophobic attitudes might well generate behavior which is counter-therapeutic, counter-productive, or renders the worker less able to be effective with homosexual clients. It follows that the client would then be hindered in his or her ability to develop and to progress as a human being. If it is demonstrated that homophobic attitudes do exist among mental health professionals, we must then address the question of how effectively workers suffering from homophobia are able to serve their clients.

Homosexuals are often seen as a threat to gender-role expectations, and we can infer that mental health practitioners are subject to the same concerns in this area as the general population. In a society that values conformity, homosexuality challenges existing values. Some workers may actually feel threatened by a homosexual client, for instance, the homosexual client may awaken the worker's own homosexual feelings, and the worker may react by denigrating the homosexual client, however subtly.

There are a number of "hidden agenda items" which the professional may not have in conscious awareness, with respect to homosexuality. For example, workers who have a hidden agenda need to establish themselves as liberal can be expected to spend time in "assuring" the homosexual client that (s)he holds no negative views about homosexuality, when such discussion is not germane to the treatment needs of the client.

The female worker who needs to reinforce her own sense of desirability as a heterosexual woman may behave in a subtly seductive manner toward a male homosexual client. In 1976, Lumby found that heterosexual respondents to an attitudinal survey on homosexuality were convinced that their own sexual orientation could not be changed due to the sexual skills of a person of the same sex but they did believe that a male homosexual could become heterosexual as a result of the sexual prowess of a woman. Lumby suggests that this difference in belief reflects the "common heterosexual optimism that it is still possible to convert the sexual deviant."

Female workers who are looking for validation of their own "femininity" might be hindered in working with a "masculine" appearing lesbian, and might well project their own hidden agenda item onto the client by imparting an unspoken message which disapproves of the client's attire or demeanor.

Other expressions of homophobia which interfere with direct and open communication with clients include making comparisons in conversation between homosexuals and cripples as reflected in psychotherapy aimed at helping homosexuals "adjust to their condition"; being condescending toward homosexual clients, frequently characterized by pointing out all of the supposed lost life opportunities being homosexual carries (such as children and marriage); identifying homosexuality in an agency case conference as one of the "problems" presented by the client being discussed; not protesting when anti-homosexual jokes are told; denying one's own homosexual feelings (Clark, 1977, points out that the mental health professional who denies having homosexual feelings is akin to an analyst who denies ever dreaming); discouraging homosexual clients from disclosing their sexual orientation to family, friends and co-workers (an attitude which imposes tremendous psychic stress on the client leading a "double" life); and in any other way disconfirming or devaluing a homosexual identity.

Comparisons have often been made between homosexuals and blacks, with respect to each group's struggle to be accepted into this society. The analogy bears up in a comparison between a white mental health professional and a black client, and a non-homosexual worker and a homosexual client. If the white worker has racist attitudes and is not aware of those feelings, the worker may well compensate by behaving in a patronizing way toward the black client. Similarly, a heterosexual worker may have hidden anti-homosexual feelings, and will likely react to them in the same way as in the previous example. The white worker who has racist feelings ought not to work with black clients and, clearly, the heterosexual worker who has anti-homosexual feelings probably ought not to work with homosexual clients.

In terms of training, most mental health professionals have had some training in working with racial and ethnic minority groups. In some states, such training is mandatory prior to being licensed. Presently an assembly bill is pending before the California legislature requiring 13 contact hours in cross-cultural issues for all therapists seeking a new or renewed license. Few professionals have had specific training in working with sexual minorities and no such training is required for licensure in any state, although California has a "human sexuality" training requirement for new and renewing therapists.

A fairly common phenomenon found in psychiatric hospitals is a considerable amount of anxiety in those staff members who work with severely disturbed patients. This anxiety is frequently activated by a deep unconscious fear of being insane. Such anxiety makes it necessary for workers to create the kind of climate in which they can assure themselves that they are sufficiently different from the patients as to be able to think of themselves as being normal, "not crazy." The need to create such a climate is the hidden agenda in this situation. The fear of being homosexual is also a deep, often unconscious, fear aroused in heterosexuals when they are in close proximity to homosexuals. This fear, known as homophobia, can be expressed in a variety of ways, through jokes, slurs or the more subtle manifestations of this fear mentioned earlier. The need to establish oneself clearly as a heterosexual and the need to create the distinct separation between the sexual orientations is the "hidden agenda."

The crux of the problem, then, relates to that intrapsychic material with which the worker may not be in touch. The limited amount of empirical evidence available suggests that those agendae can be identified and, with sufficient training, eliminated. It is not surprising that homophobic attitudes can be found among mental health practitioners, even homosexual ones. Most mental health professionals include training in the psychoanalytic tradition in their education and, even in the light of contemporary psychoanalytic thinking, are likely to view homosexual people as immature, arrested in terms of sexual development, or neurotic by definition. It is likely that such an attitude will be conveyed to clients and negatively affect the self esteem of homosexual clients. Homophobia is a prejudice which, among mental health practitioners, breeds and causes counterproductive behavior with clients.

Few systematic efforts to measure homophobia among mental health practitioners have been made, although the subject of homophobia has been discussed in professional literature for many years (Gorer, 1948; Hoffman, 1968; Hooker, 1965; Weinberg, 1972). The professional literature reflects a wide disparity between attitudes toward liberalizing laws governing behavior among consenting adults and those attitudes and values which influence the interaction between clients and mental health professionals.[1]

COMMONLY HELD BELIEFS

In order to construct a questionnaire which would reflect contemporary thinking with respect to homosexuality, the researchers first reviewed the literature covering various attitudinal surveys and studies, both among the general population and the mental health professions. Some commonly held beliefs emerged from that review.

1. Homosexuals of both sexes have a history of disturbed relationships with either or both parents.
2. Homosexuality is a neurotic disorder.
3. Homosexuals have difficulty in achieving close relationships.
4. Homosexuals are sexually promiscuous.
5. Male homosexuals have unusually close relationships with their mothers.
6. Homosexuals adjust poorly psychologically.
7. Homosexuals use drugs and alcohol to a greater degree than non-homosexuals.
8. Male homosexuals tend to be child abusers.
9. Homosexuality can be reversed with adequate psychotherapeutic intervention.

10. Homosexuality represents an arrested state of psychosexual development.

With respect to the origin of these beliefs, Weinberg (1972) asserts that homophobia arises from the Judeo-Christian religious taboo against homosexuality, the secret fear of being homosexual, repressed envy of the perceived ease in life of homosexuals, the view of homosexuality as a threat to societal and familial values and the re-awakening of fears of death caused by homosexuals often being persons without children.

If, however, the origin of these beliefs cannot be attributed to cultural myths and taboos, then they ought to be found in science, with empirical evidence. Morin (1977) points out that early psychological writings on homosexuality do not document empirical research. Rather, he observes, most of the writings are generalizations based on an analyst's construction of his or her client's reconstruction of childhood and following from idiosyncratic variations of a psychoanalytic perspective. The first empirical studies to address the question of whether or not homosexuality, per se, was indicative of psychopathology were devised in the late 1950s by Evelyn Hooker. Though she demonstrated that trained clinicians could not differentiate the sexual orientation of homosexual nonpatients from that of non-homosexuals who were also non-patients through the use of standard projective techniques, Hooker's findings have been generally ignored in psychoanalytic writings since their publication.

To further the construction of a questionnaire which would reflect a tension between the commonly held beliefs and empirical considerations, a second literature review was conducted to determine whether or not there is evidence to support those commonly held beliefs. The only belief for which there is empirical evidence is that homosexuals do use drugs and alcohol to a greater degree than do non-homosexuals. None of the other beliefs stands up to scientific inquiry.

For example, Bieber's (1962) view that homosexuality is a neurotic condition characterized by undue anxiety, a view shared by many contemporary professionals, is challenged by research in which there is no difference between homosexuals and heterosexuals on tests designed to measure anxiety (Siegelman, 1972). Studies comparing the childhood memories of male homosexuals and heterosexuals do not support the commonly held belief that male homosexuals have unusually close-binding relationships with their mothers (Bene, 1965). The image of the male homosexual as child molester dims in the light of research confirming that more than 95% of reported child molestation is perpetrated by adult males on minor females (U.S. Department of Health, Education and Welfare, National Center on Child Abuse and Neglect, 1977). The prevalent view of lesbians as being poorly adjusted psychologically is questioned by research which found that lesbian and non-lesbian groups of women did not differ in total psychological adjustment as measured by scales on the MMPI, nor as evaluated by expert blind raters using the MMPI profiles (Oberstone and Sukonek, 1976).

The literature is not wanting for reports on the successful reversal of the sexual orientation of homosexuals (Hadden, 1968; Truax and Tourney, 1970, 1971; Johnsgard and Schumacher, 1970; Covi, 1972, and others). These reports detail not only the successful outcome possible in such treatment, but also point out the importance of such interventions. Singer and Fischer (1967) observe that no group of patients "so clearly reveals such pathological gender distortion as does an all homosexual group." Nobler (1972) cautions against the detrimental impact of "various homosexual freedom groups," whose attitudes are "very confusing to the men in the group . . . they are torn between thinking of themselves as an oppressed minority fighting for acceptance of homosexuality and what they are striving for in the group . . . many persons who could be helped therapeutically are deterred from seeking help."

Rogers (1975) et al., comment in part, "we are concerned with, and question the ethics of, approaches in which the deception as to the goals of therapy is utilized as a technique to gain commitment on the part of the homosexual to treatment. A distressing practice is the treatment approach of some therapists of offering the patient no treatment alternative except that of achieving a heterosexual pattern of adjustment."

With respect to substance abuse, Clark (1977) notes that "the gay person is likely to be tempted to dull the pain that surfaces now and again through misuse of drugs and alcohol. . .the use of alcohol is reinforced since gay bars are one of the few community approved meeting places for gay people.

THE STUDY

An initial pool of more than 200 items, based on the literature reviews noted, was submitted to a panel of three independent judges, who evaluated items both in terms of relevance to the research topic and in terms of adequate measurement of the identified aspect of the study. In addition to the 23 demographic variables,[2] the study was designed to measure three distinct aspects of homophobia: the first area to be considered was that of stereotype thinking, that is, whether the respondent tends to view homosexuals in terms of "caricatures," such as male homosexuals as effeminate and female homosexuals as masculine; the second area for consideration was that of psychopathology, that is, to what degree homosexuality in and of itself was seen as indicative of mental disturbance; the third area of investigation was "general" homophobia, that is, whether or not respondents might demonstrate a certain liberal kind of thinking in some areas but express their own personal unwillingness to socialize with, live next door to, or otherwise be in close proximity to homosexuals.

In order to achieve consistency in language, respondents were informed that homosexuality refers to erotic, affectional and/or sexual preference for persons of the same gender. Further, since many women refer to themselves as homosexual or gay while others prefer the term lesbian, the language in the instrument reflected these differences. In each questionnaire item referring to males, the phrase "homosexual/gay" was used, while references to females were termed "homosexual/lesbian." Respondents were mental health professionals from various agencies throughout the greater Los Angeles area. For the purposes of this study, a mental health professional was defined as anyone having client or patient contact, and holding at least a master's degree in one of the behavioral sciences; workers with a lesser degree, such as a BSW, having significant client or patient contact as a regular part of their duties; and graduate students and interns who were assigned to an agency as a specific part of their training. One reason for including the latter two categories was to determine whether lack of professional training may result in differing attitudes toward homosexuality. Other data with respect to specific duties were also gathered.[3]

Eight discrete populations were sampled, five of them from large, publicly-funded agencies and three private, non-sectarian family service agencies. The sampling procedure was based on access to agencies, thus, a probability sampling was not possible, nor was randomization of respondents. This accidental, non-probability sampling, which yields low external validity, represents the major weakness of the study. Nonetheless, there is considerable value in establishing the base for further research in this area, if specific patterns of response emerged in this study.

Participants included 41% direct service practitioners, 25% combined supervision and service providers, 20% interns and graduate students and 11% paraprofessionals. The vast majority was employed in publicly funded organizations (84%) and approximately 60% were female.

Non-demographic items were set up on a Likert-type scale, offering a range of responses indicating level of agreement or disagreement ranging from 1 to 7 with 4 being considered to be a neutral response. Allowing 7 degrees of response increased reliability and provided more precise information on the respondent's opinion per issue, item for item. As noted earlier, there were three specific "sub-scales," though five general areas were at issue, including the relationship between the respondent's sexual orientation and treatment goals; the effect of intervention strategy on treatment outcome; psychodynamic formulation and speculation regarding the etiology of homosexuality; perception of stereotypically homosexual behavior; and statements about homosexuality of a very general nature with social implications vis-à-vis public policy.

There were also four items at the end of the questionnaire which were not on a Likert-type scale. These items included two "forced choice" responses and a request for respondents to locate themselves on the Kinsey Scale (Kinsey, et al., 1948). Responses to these items provided the most interesting findings of the study.

RESULTS AND DISCUSSION

As noted above, the most telling findings emerged from the last four items in the questionnaire, those non "Likert-type" items, which asked respondents several specific questions about themselves in relation to their own sexual orientation. Respondents were asked to locate themselves on the Kinsey Scale. Those who rated themselves in the upper brackets of the Scale seemed to perceive homosexuals/gays in the least stereotypic terms. That is an expected result, since they are self-identified homosexuals/gays. Predictably, those who identify as exclusively heterosexual perceived homosexuals/gays in more stereotypic terms. What is particularly interesting to note, however, is that those who placed themselves in the "bisexual" position on the Scale are very close in "stereotype score" to the "exclusive heterosexuals."

The same dichotomy in viewpoint appears at the upper and lower ends of the Scale on items related to psychopathology. However, those who ranked themselves closest to "bisexual" seem the least certain as to whether homosexuals/gays are clinically disturbed.

Four of the 140 respondents did not answer the question, "are you homosexual/gay?" Of those who did respond to this question, five identified as homosexual/gay. These five respondents rated homosexuals/gays as not being clinically disturbed. Of the remaining answers, 117 persons said that they were not homosexual/gay, while five persons selected the response choice, "none of your business," and six selected the answer, "I'm not sure yet." These latter six respondents got the highest scores in terms of perceiving homosexuals/gays as most clinically disturbed.

The relationship between one's own sexual orientation and the way one views homosexuality and bisexuality is an area in which little research has been conducted. Goffman (1963) posited that the person who carries a visible "stigma sign," such as the label "homosexual," is reduced from a whole and usual person to a discounted one. Thus, homosexuals whose sexuality has been revealed join other large groups who face social rejection and discrimination because of their condition (poor, insane, terminally ill, etc.).

Ullman and Krasner (1969) observed that people who are deemed deviant in general, receive social reinforcement only for the limited range of behaviors which are compatible with the particular label they carry. They note that a "stigmatizing label, such as homosexual, imparts a generalized negative halo that overwhelms all other personal characteristics and predefines the reactions of others to all subsequent behavior."

If the label predefines not only the reactions of others, but imparts a particular aura which overshadows other characteristics, then it is likely that most people will attempt to block or repress the development of a homosexual identity. This concept is supported by Davidson and Wilson (1973), who point out that the development of a homosexual identity is blocked, not only by a lack of information, but also by prejudice. They state that this category has too great a stigma attached to it and, therefore, the development of that identity is avoided. Further, an individual who sees homosexuality as a problem in one's self or in others will likely see a need to avoid that identity, or to change it if one is already homosexual. When "one learns what a homosexual is at a cognitive level, one also learns what a homosexual is at an affective level, i.e., bad, tense, feminine, static, passive and changeable."

In fact, other writers have suggested that society attempts to block the development of a homosexual identity (Dank, 1971; Hedblom, 1973) in two ways:

1. A homosexual identity cannot occur in an environment where the cognitive category of homosexuality does not exist.
2. When the category does exist and is closely associated with mental illness, there will be an avoidance of such self-definition.

In effect, all of the writers from Goffman to Hedblom are saying that a person in conflict is not likely to identify with, or to feel good about, that which (s)he associates with mental illness, or perceives as stigmatized or "bad." Inferentially, from the scores of those respondents who were either not sure about their sexual orientation or were conflicted in the self-rating, it appears that they are not only experiencing uncertainty about their sexual orientation per se, but they may also be unable to tolerate the idea of their own identity being associated with stereotypic images of homosexuality and the social stigma that label still carries.

Other findings include where people reside in the greater Los Angeles area being positively correlated with high homophobia and stereotype scores; where people were born in the United States is similarly positively correlated. As noted earlier, these results are not generalized to all mental health professionals because of sampling problems, nonetheless, it is noteworthy that people born in more "conservative" areas of the United States do appear to have more homophobic attitudes than those born in so-called "liberal" areas. The same trend was found in terms of where people lived in and around Los Angeles, ranging from "liberal" areas to more "conservative" neighborhoods.

Social workers achieved the highest homophobia scores, while psychologists were found to be the least homophobic. A number of explanations might account for these differences. For example, the issue of dealing with the gay and lesbian client population has been a topic of much concern and high visibility among psychologists for several years. The Association of Gay Psychologists has pressed for reform among their colleagues, psychology journals have published numerous articles dealing with homosexuality and most psychology conferences have presentations discussing lesbian and gay clients. The issue of homosexuality has had little visibility among social workers until just recently. The lesbian and gay task forces both in the National Association of Social Work and the Council on Social Work Education have been in existence a relatively short period of time and efforts to organize the Association of Lesbian and Gay Social Workers have met with limited success. Few articles have been published in social work journals about treating lesbian and gay clients, social work conferences have just recently begun to address the concerns of this client population and most of the social workers responding to the questionnaire in this study indicated that they do not believe they know many, if any, lesbian or gay people.

It follows then, that those respondents who are aware that they know homosexuals give fewer homophobic responses and see homosexuals less in terms of stereotypes and as less clinically sick. Most of the literature on prejudice speaks to the fears and misconceptions about the unknown.

Married respondents saw homosexuals/gays as being significantly more clinically disturbed than did single respondents, and also saw homosexuals/gays in more stereotypic terms. It seems reasonable that we tend to identify with people most like ourselves and may see people who are different from us as less healthy than we are. Thus, we may avoid contact with them only further reinforcing our misconceptions and prejudices about them. Unmarried people may have more contact with a wider variety of people, thereby having the opportunity to test out some of the commonly held beliefs mentioned earlier. Also, as Weinberg points out, homophobia is caused, in part, by envy of a perceived ease in life of homosexuals/gay people. Married people may view homosexuals as irresponsible, since many homosexuals/gays do not have children and are seen as being free to indulge in more recreational pursuits. Also, the reality that marriage may lead to procreation might well impact on people's views about homosexuality. Parenting is a highly emotionally charged role. Although many can be tolerant of "deviant" behavior in others, the idea of one's own children identifying as homosexual could cause the issue to become clouded. If one says, in effect, "homosexuality is all right, but I would not want my child to become one," this message will necessarily be transmitted to their own children and likely to clients, especially those clients who are children or adolescents.

There was also a statistically significant correlation between "stereotype score" and the greater number of clients "suspected" of being homosexual/gay. It follows that, if one tends to see homosexuals in terms of stereotype, then the "feminine" appearing male will be suspected of being homosexual and the androgynous female will be suspected of being a lesbian.

The religious values of the family of origin appear to have significant impact on how "sick" gay people are perceived, lending further credence to Weinberg's argument that homophobia is inculcated early in life, and further makes viable the concept introduced earlier that attitudes toward homosexuals have gone through a kind of circular metamorphosis from religious injunctions to law to mental health theories.

The numerous variables considered in this study produced a wide variety of findings.[4]

IMPLICATIONS FOR PRACTICE

The findings of this study demonstrate the need for social work education in order to dispel those myths and stereotypes about homosexual/gay people, which persist despite the lack of empirical evidence to support them. Social workers seem to have limited access to factual information about a sizeable client population.

Since people who are aware that they know gays and lesbians are less homophobic, see gays and lesbians as less sick, and do not see lesbians and gays in terms of stereotypes as noted, an aggressive recruitment program of lesbian and gay students by graduate schools of social work seems very much in order. Also, making a general outreach to the lesbian and gay population would enable social workers to widen their range of awareness about homosexuality. Although most social work graduate schools have added a "human sexuality" course and more can be expected to add such

courses as state licensing laws governing mental health professionals demand completion of such courses, these classes often present
a cursory treatment of homosexuality, usually only including a
film depicting specific sex acts involving homosexuals. Also,
other studies have confirmed that most professionals employed full
time by agencies tend to seek new information within the context
of the work setting. Therefore, it is important that agencies make
accurate information about homosexuality available to its employees.

One point to consider in the course content of a program is the
importance of removing "homosexuality" from its status as one
portion of a "human sexuality" program. The rationale for this rec-
ommendation is that homosexuality ought not to be presented to
trainees in a clinical context; such a presentation furthers the mistaken impression that homosexuality is an aberration. Also, one of
the difficulties in understanding the needs of a lesbian and gay client population is due, in part, to the oversexualizing of the image
of this group of people. What homosexuals do sexually is not very
different from what heterosexuals do. It is the other, widely varied, aspects of gay lifestyles which the non-gay mental health
worker needs to know in order to serve this client population effectively, not what they do in bed. It is important not to limit instruc-
tion on homosexuality to the mechanics of sex, and it is crucial to
go beyond showing an explicit sex film as an adequate presentation of the lives of some 20 million Americans.

In planning a training program on homosexuality and gay lifestyles, a number of factors should be considered, including criteria
for the selection of individuals to present such a program; adequate
evaluation of the program design as well as the specific course
content; and participative experience for those attending such a
program.

Often, in presentations about homosexuality, volunteers from
local gay activist organizations are solicited to speak to issues regarding homosexuality, about which they might know very little.
Persons being considered to deliver such programs should have adequate professional credentials and a documented history in human
relations training of a comparable nature. Such professionals
should have a reputation for credibility, reliability and effectiveness in past training projects.

A well-designed training program would include three major
components: *factual information, theoretical material* and *partici-*

pative experience for those attending such a program. Specific topics would include information about what homosexuality is, what is known about its cause and incidence; a discussion of why prejudice against the homosexual minority exists, and how the major sources of that prejudice have operated to perpetuate the problem; a description of the contemporary gay and lesbian world; and a presentation of myths and stereotypes regarding lesbians and gay men with accurate information regarding each point.

Further course content would include a consideration of homophobia, its etiology and symptomology; religious issues of concern to lesbians and gays; love relationships and coupling in the lesbian and gay community; lesbian and gay culture, history and humor; difficulties encountered in the "coming out" or disclosure process; lesbian and gay parents, children and lesbian and gay family relationships; ageing in the lesbian and gay world; legal issues of relevance to lesbians and gay men; civil rights issues around differential treatment under the law; and films about the wide variety of lesbian and gay lifestyles which depict relevant material that does not define gay people only in terms of sexual activity.

Sexual problems of lesbians and gay men is a legitimate area of training for mental health professionals usually ignored in most presentations, and could include a discussion of sexual dysfunction among lesbians and gay men, sex therapy with lesbian and gay clients and recent developments in sexual surrogate treatment of lesbians and gays who have sexual problems.

Guidelines for clinical intervention with lesbian and gay clients warrant considerable attention in a training program for social workers, including theoretical material postulating gay-oriented, gay-supportive therapy and case histories addressing areas of concern in arriving at theoretical formulations.[5]

Role playing, guided fantasies, encounter and other techniques might be employed to enhance the participative experience of those taking such a course. There should always be presentations by lesbians and gay men in any training program about homosexuality, since homosexuals have much to offer in terms of de-mythologizing their image in this society.

Participants in such a program should also have access to resource lists of the nearly 2000 formally organized gay and lesbian groups within the United States, in order that they might more fully appreciate and acquaint themselves with the rich diversity of the lesbian and gay population in America, and so that they will be aware of resources to which they might refer lesbian and gay clients.

It is certainly important to recognize that, by definition, social workers often see a troubled population. Expanded awareness of the broader range of lesbian and gay peoples' lives is essential to workers' knowledge base. Also, individual acceptance of the personal set of biases brought to any profession might help clinicians and other social workers to discover that, all things being equal, it might be best not to assume the ability to treat all clients, and to consider referring lesbian and gay clients to qualified lesbian and gay therapists, where indicated.

Lesbian and gay affirming psychotherapy posits a theoretical orientation for mental health practitioners:

1. Homosexuality is a natural variant in the expression of human sexuality, which is statistically less common than the heterosexual variant, and should not be regarded as a "spoiled identity."
2. Adult homosexuality occurs because of a pattern of development that is unique to each individual. The pattern is influenced by genetic and prenatal factors, hormonal factors, social learning with modifying factors, including personal sexual experience, the reaction of self and others to sexual experience, the fantasies one has by which (s)he tries out possibilities for self, and the cultural factors in the society in which one lives.
3. Homosexuality consists of intrapsychic experiences involving erotic, affectional thoughts, feelings, fantasies about individuals of the same sex, and/or interpersonal behaviors which are expressive of those erotic feelings of attraction for persons of the same gender.
4. The majority of homosexuals are emotionally healthy individuals who are stable, productive, who like themselves, and who have fulfilling relationships.
5. Same sex coupling is a valid expression of the partners' need to give and to receive love in a long term, intimate relationship. There are ambiguities in the bonding process, but such relationships do occur and are possible for those who will work at such relationships.
6. All lesbian and gay people suffer oppression at some level, from the private, self-inflicted kind, to that involving actual

threat and/or loss of dignity, of livelihood, of family support, of civil liberties and, often, life itself.

Berzon and Clark (1974) developed a series of therapeutic guidelines for professionals working with lesbian and gay clients and Clark (1977) points out that the training and "retraining" of professionals should include specific experiential, as well as didactic, material.[6]

As observed earlier, this report discusses partial findings only, as the volume of data is so great as to require more space for reportage. Also, some data are being analyzed presently; one such piece of data is the 9-item scale which emerged and which, unlike previous efforts to construct a valid homophobia scale which failed to meet minimum Guttman Scalogram requirements (Nie et al., 1970), these nine items achieved a Guttman coefficient of reproducibility of .96. The scale is presently being retested, and there is considerable optimism that a valid homophobia scale may yet emerge.

NOTES

1. For a discussion of the previous research on homophobia, the reader is referred to the *Journal of Homosexuality,* 2, 1, 1976, p. 39-47, Homophobia: The Quest For a Valid Scale, Lumby, M.E.

2. Variables include year of birth, sex, marital status, number of children, present living arrangement, racial or ethnic identification, birth state and description of population, present zip code, educational degrees earned, area of study plus year and location, parents' religious preference and frequency of church attendance, respondent's religious preference and frequency of church attendance, social class of family of origin, income level, professional identification and socialization patterns. Each of these is considered important to the findings, since the study aimed, in part, to determine how, singly or in combination, these factors influence an individual's attitude toward homosexuality.

3. These data included job title and description of duties, agency funding sources (private or public, sectarian or non-sectarian), service function and size of agency, employment status including length of time and position, monthly volume of clients, number of known homosexual/gay/lesbian clients seen, number of clients the worker suspected might be homosexual/gay/lesbian and the number of same sex couples currently in treatment.

4. A copy of all of the findings of the study is available from the author.

5. An example of such relevant research is: Chalus, G.A., An Evaluation of the Validity of the Freudian Theory of Paranoia, *Journal of Homosexuality,* 3, 2, Winter, 1977, p. 171-185; and Psychotherapy and Homosexuality, *Journal of Homosexuality,* Fall, 1982.

6. These 12 guidelines may be found in Clark, Don, *Loving Someone Gay,* Celestial Arts, Millbrae, California, 1977 and Berzon, B. and Clark, D., "Twelve Therapeutic Guidelines," 1974, paper delivered at Association for Humanistic Psychology, New Orleans, Louisiana.

REFERENCES

Bene, E. (1965) On the Genesis of Male Homosexuality: An Attempt at Clarifying the Role of the Parents. *British Journal of Psychiatry,* 111: 803.

Berzon, B. The New Gay Therapy, Unpublished paper, 1976.

Berzon, B. and Clark, D. Twelve Therapeutic Guidelines. Paper delivered at Association for Humanistic Psychology Annual Meeting, New Orleans, 1974.

Bieber, I. *Homosexuality,* Basic Books, New York, 1962.

Clark, D. *Loving Someone Gay.* Celestial Arts, Millbrae, CA., 1977.

Covi, J. A Group Psychotherapy Approach to the Treatment of Neurotic Symptoms in Male and Female Patients of Homosexual Preference, *Psychotherapy and Psychosomatics,* 1972, *20,* 176-180.

Dank, B. Coming Out in the Gay World, *Psychiatry,* 1971, *34,* 180-197.

Davison, C.C., and Wilson, T.G. Attitudes of Behavior Therapists Toward Homosexuality, *Behavior Therapy,* 1973, 4, 686-696.

Freedman, M. Gays Function Better than Straights, *Psychology Today,* March, 1975.

Goffman, I. *Stigma,* Prentice-Hall, 1963, Englewood Cliffs, N.J.

Gorer, G. *The American People,* W.W. Norton Co., New York, 1948.

Hadden, S.B. Treatment of Homosexuality by Individual and Group Psychotherapy, *American Journal of Psychiatry,* 1958, 114, 810-815.

Hedblom, J.H. Dimensions of Lesbian Sexual Experience, *Archives of Sexual Behavior,* 1973, 2, 4, 329-341.

Hoffman, M. *The Gay World: Male Homosexuality and the Social Creation of Evil,* 1972, New York.

Hooker, E. Male Homosexuals and Their Worlds, 1965, in J. Marmor (Ed.) *Sexual Inversion,* Basic Books, New York.

Karr, R. Homosexual Labelling: An Experimental Study. Paper presented at Western Psychological Association Convention, 1975.

Kinsey, A.C. and Pomeroy, W.B. and Martin, C.E., 1948, *Sexual Behavior in the Human Male,* Saunders, Philadelphia, Pa.

Lauritsen, J. and Thorstad, D. *The Early Homosexual Rights Movement, (1864-1935),* Times Change Press, New York, 1974.

Morin, S.F. Attitudes Toward Homosexuality and Social Distance. Paper presented at the American Psychological Association meeting Chicago, 1975.

Nobler, H. Group Therapy with Male Homosexuals, *Comparative Group Studies,* 1972, *3,* 161-178.

Oberstone, A.K. and Sukoneck, H. Psychological Adjustment and Lifestyle of Single Lesbians and Single Heterosexual Women, *Psychology of Women Quarterly, 1, 2,* 1976.

Rogers, C. and Roback, H. and McKee, E. and Calhoun, D. Group Psychotherapy with Homosexuals: A Review, *International Journal of Group Psychotherapy,* 1975.

Selltiz, C. Wrightsman, L.S. and Cook, S.W. *Research Methods in Social Relations,* Rinehart and Wilson, New York, 1976.

Siegelman, M. Adjustment of Male Homosexuals and Heterosexuals, *Archives of Sexual Behavior, 2,* 9, 1972.

Singer, M. and Fischer, R. Group Psychotherapy of Male Homosexuals by a Male and Female Co-therapy Team, *International Journal of Group Psychotherapy, 17,* 44-52, 1967.

Traux, R.A., Moeller, W.S. and Tourney, G. The Medical Approach to Male Homosexuality, *Journal of the Iowa Medical Society, 60,* 397-403, 1970.

Weinberg, G. *Society and the Healthy Homosexual,* Anchor Books, Garden City, New York, 1972.

Teaching Social Workers to Meet the Needs of the Homosexually Oriented

Harvey L. Gochros

Almost a decade ago I wrote "Teaching More or Less Straight Social Work Students to be Helpful to More or Less Gay People."[1] The article was written at a critical point in the gay and lesbian movement. The radicalism of the '60s was showing its effects. The Stonewall episode—in which gays in a New York City Greenwich Village bar fought back against police harrassment—became a symbol of a growing assertiveness by gays and lesbians and demands for an end to their oppression. For the first time television and movies were beginning to recognize that homosexually oriented men and women existed, and portrayed them as three dimensional non-neurotic human beings.

Reflecting this shift in public opinion, in 1973 the American Psychiatric Association voted to no longer consider homosexuality, per se, as an illness. A number of State legislatures slowly fell in line in repealing state laws against homosexual acts between consenting adults in private.

In the midst of all this, social work education was catching up with social work practice by introducing content on human sexuality—including, with varying degrees of caution—discussions of homosexuality as a common and non-pathological phenomenon.[2]

The years since the publication of that article may be seen as a time of consolidation. The radicalism and the furor of the '60s and early '70s seem far distant and almost difficult to comprehend. The effects of the previous decades are certainly still with us. We have profited from the chaos of the past. But change is slower now. Most Americans have less conviction that abrupt social

The author expresses his appreciation to Wendell Ricketts for his assistance in the preparation of this manuscript.

137

changes are possible or even desirable. We are mellower both as citizens and as social workers.

Indeed, if a trend can be detected in our current attitudes toward sex in general and homosexuality in particular, it would seem to be toward conservatism. "Sexual freedom" seems no longer to be a rallying cry, and the preoccupation with optimal genital joy, with its associated band of professional sexual plumbers sound strangely old-fashioned. National magazines feature articles proclaiming "Is Sex Dead?" ("Not Exactly, But it Ain't What it Used to Be!") and "The End of Sex" ("Isn't it Time We Stopped Thinking About Sex and Started Thinking About Something Else?")

The "something else" seems to be relationships. I believe we will look back upon the '80s as a period in which there was a resurgence of interest in love. The recently published research of McWhirter and Matteson, for example, focuses on the stages of development and coping strategies of male couples. They found that after the first year or so of a relationship, gay couples are bound together much more by affection than by sexual interests.[3] The rediscovery of intimacy has therefore had a profound impact on the perceptions of people of all sexual orientations. The epidemics of herpes and AIDS may have been a contributing factor. Also, economic depression inevitably draws people together. Perhaps it might even be a response to our increasingly "high-tech" society. Whatever the underlying factors, relationship and commitment seem to be eclipsing the search for ultimate sexual fulfillment in the lives of many people.

These reminiscences and attempts to quickly survey the current sexual scene are presented as a preface to the first point I would like to make regarding teaching social workers about homosexuality: The study of sex-related behaviors is basically the study of individual and collective attitudes about those behaviors. These attitudes vary from culture to culture and over time. Therefore, to understand problems related to homosexuality, social workers must first understand not only individuals' attitudes about their own homosexuality, but the attitudes of those who influence or are influenced by them, including those within the social systems that impact upon them. Furthermore, social workers must also examine and perhaps re-examine their own attitudes about homosexual feelings and behaviors in themselves and others.

In the classes I teach for social work students, and the workshops I present for social work practitioners, I find no other sex-related topic (except, perhaps, incest and adult masturbation) which still provokes as much interest and at the same time confusion and discomfort as homosexuality. This, despite the aforementioned "sexual revolution." The major tasks of those who teach social workers about homosexuality is to overcome this discomfort, explore sources of prejudice, replace stereotypes with knowledge, and instill a willingness to provide effective social work services to those who are more or less homosexually oriented.

The remainder of this chapter will review some of the ways I have found useful to approach these tasks and to help students think about homosexuality.

SOURCES OF DISCOMFORT

A primary function of social work courses in sex-related problems is to explore and understand the sources of students' discomfort related to sexual matters and decrease it, allowing them to develop greater objectivity and a more "casual" approach to their clients' sexual behavior. This would seem to be a prerequisite of learning to be of help. A number of factors contribute to discomfort about homosexual behavior. These sources are similar to those experienced by many in the general public. Understanding their *own* discomfort may therefore help students understand the discomfort of those with whom they will have contact in their professional practice and those who may contribute to the difficulties encountered by those who are homosexually oriented. These factors have provided a focus for a number of learning experiences for social work students. Some of these factors are discussed below:

PERSONAL EXPERIENCE

A substantial number of students have had homosexual experiences or fantasies in their past or present, although they may not label themselves as gay. While a minority of social work students (and practitioners) are exclusively homosexual in their behavior, and even fewer have "come out," a larger number have at some time or other, for a greater or lesser period of time, engaged in sexual relationships with other people of their own sex. An even greater number have fantasied such relationships.[4] Such fantasies often provoke guilt and shame in the people who experience them. They may rarely be shared with others who may or may not also have similar wishes or fantasies. Such experiences may indeed contribute to both discomfort (fear of revelation and exploration behind this door which most have been taught to keep closed) and, at the same time curiosity ("what are these people like who act out these fantasies, and what can I learn about myself"?) While the prevailing attitudes toward homosexual orientation as an illness have changed radically in recent years, there still may be an apprehension on the part of some students that course content will confirm that image of homosexual feelings and so adjudicate them as sick. Further, some students (especially men) may fear that showing acceptance and understanding of homosexuality or even interest in problems related to homosexuality may call into question their own sexual orientation or start them on a path they would prefer not enter. Whether or not students have identified themselves as gay, they may have considerable discomfort with any gayness they perceive in themselves or any gayness others might conceivably perceive in them.

THE OPPRESSION/PATHOLOGY DILEMMA

Homosexuality poses a dilemma for social work. The profession has evolved with a dual tradition of overcoming oppression on one hand and "curing" pathology on the other. If we try to cure (read: convert) homosexuals are we merely supporting the oppression based on the reproductive bias?[5] And if we fight oppression and leave the homosexually oriented alone are we ultimately ignoring their "sickness?"

Tully and Albro[6] have called homosexuality a "social worker's imbroglio" and describe the social worker's moral dilemma when faced with a sexual revolution which includes increased acceptance of homosexuality; conflicting significantly with the family-centered values that social work has traditionally upheld. At the same time, negative attitudes toward the homosexually oriented are still strong and widespread.[7]

The "pathological" view of homosexuality pervades much of the mental health field. There has been some movement to accept homosexuality as one variation of the need for love and sexual expression. As noted earlier, the 1973 decision of the American Psychiatric Association to remove homosexuality per se from the *Diagnostic and Statistical Manual* represented some tangible progress in separating homosexuality from a "disease" model to which it had been relegated for so long. However, a survey of behavior therapists published that same year revealed that 13 percent would consider the use of aversive behavioral techniques to eliminate homosexuality *even in cases in which the clients did not want to change.*[8] Even Masters and Johnson, who serve as role models for those in the helping professions who work with sex-related problems, assert in a recent book that while homosexuality is learned and not intrinsically a "disease," they can effectively reorient homosexually oriented individuals in a relatively short treatment regimen.[9] Current brochures advertising the travelling workshops presented by Masters and Johnson and their staff feature sessions on the treatment of "ego-dystonic" homosexuality.

While books and articles describing homosexuality as a disease are becoming rarer, an attitude still pervades much of professional literature which portrays homosexuality as, if not an illness, at least a misfortune. Garfinkel and Morin report that clinicians often lack awareness of the adaptive advantages and potential satisfactions of gay life styles, and generally believe that the homosexually oriented are destined to lead difficult and unsatisfying lives.[10]

Donald Brown, in an otherwise helpful article falls into a typical, "heterosexual bias" when he writes "Because of the additional problems associated with homosexuality, an individual having complete freedom of choice would probably be better off as a heterosexual."[11] The basic message of this approach is that homosexuality is at best "second best" and wherever possible, those leaning in a homosexual direction would be well advised to bend the other way. This attitude is behind the conversion therapy frenzy of the last decade in which many behaviorists attempted to help their clients "go straight." Students may be helped to understand the oppressiveness underlying such an approach by the analogy of efforts directed toward a racial minority group to help them look, think, act and sound more "white" because their lives would be "easier" that way.

If not treated as sick or second best, homosexual orientations can be oppressed by being ignored. Bernie Zilbergeld in his widely acclaimed book *Male Sexuality*[12] virtually overlooks homosexual feelings, activities and relationships. He implies that male sexuality is essentially *heterosexuality* and reinforces the idea that homosexual feelings are outside the range of "normal" sexual expression. This idea is shared by many students, faculty, practitioners, writers and researchers alike despite the fact that at least one out of four people has had at least incidental homosexual experiences in their lives.

Thus the social worker must integrate conflicting social values, religious beliefs, laws and clinical traditions as well as convictions about human rights. The task of social work educators is to help explore and evaluate each of these factors as they bear upon the student's development of a professional stance on homosexuality.

In order to better understand the issues and problems associated with homosexuality, the student must first be helped to explore evolving ideas about homosexuality which depart from conventional wisdom. These ideas can be organized around the concepts of reification and bifurcation of sexual orientation and the consequences of the invisibility of homosexuality.

THE REIFICATION AND BIFURCATION OF SEXUAL ORIENTATION

It can be argued that there are no homosexuals. Indeed, it can also be argued that there are no heterosexuals. The labels heterosexual and homosexual are relatively new, as is the idea that people can be categorized by their sexual preference. Until the late 19th century, when the terms homosexual and heterosexual were invented, terms like "sodomy," "buggery," "pederasty," and "unnatural vices" were used to describe criminal *acts* of which, presumably, anyone could be guilty. Since then, "homosexuality" emerged as a total personal identity. According to Focault "The sodomite had been a temporary aberration; the homosexual was now a species."[13]

The idea that people can be classified by their sexual gender preferences is a reification: that is, taking a *concept* (e.g., sexual preferences) and treating the total person as if he or she were permeated with that quality; indeed he or she *is* that quality. Thus a person is not defined as someone who to a greater or lesser extent in certain situations sexually and/or emotionally is attracted to a person or persons of their own sex, but rather they themselves are defined as homosexuals. This process is not unlike the efforts of Senator Joseph McCarthy in the 1950s to define certain people as *being* communists if certain of their behaviors or even ideas met his criteria.

Related to the concept of reification is the concept of bifurcation in which phenomena are perceived as existing only in either of two opposite forms: black or white, night or day. Bifurcation is a common approach of the medical model in viewing human behavior (abnormal or normal, psychotic or neurotic, healthy or sick). It is not surprising therefore that our view of sexual preferences should be bifurcated: gay or straight, homosexual or heterosexual.

However, people do not divide reality into these two pidgeon-holes. As Kinsey noted people do not divide neatly into "sheep and goats." Their sexual interests fall along a continuum which can vary over time. Yet this sexual dichotimization persists even among sex educators and counselors, despite Kinsey's elaborate (if flawed) conceptualization of a continuum of human sexual response, with over a quarter of the adult population something other than exclusively heterosexual or homosexual in their sexual preferences and activities.[14]

Bifurcation of sexual preference conceptualizations contributes to a tendency for even the most incidental same-sex experiences to be considered evidence of a "homosexual orientation" and encourages self and other labeling. For the many who are unsure of their commitment to one of the exclusively gay lifestyles, or who are able to respond erotically to both men and women, such labeling is inaccurate and potentially damaging.

There is much in our society and within the helping professions which maintains the reification and bifurcation of sexual orientations. W.I. Thomas noted that "If men define situations as real, they are real in their consequences."[15] Students can explore the factors which maintain this reification and bifurcation in social work and consider their hazards to social behaviors and individual social functioning.

INVISIBILITY

A major factor contributing to the problems associated with homosexuality as well as the difficulties students and practitioners encounter in relation to homosexuality is its invisibility. No other large, oppressed group is so invisible to the general public as those who are homosexually oriented. A basic concept to be presented to social work students is the vast majority of homosexually oriented adolescents, men and women are indistinguishable from those who are exclusively heterosexually oriented. Indeed, it is likely that the majority of people with some degree of homosexual orientation ultimately marry, and that many, if not most, go to their graves with few if any people in their environment knowing their interests. Wardell Pomeroy (Kinsey's chief researcher) estimated that the sexual orientations of approximately 85% of those exclusively homosexual subjects who were interviewed by Kinsey's researchers were undetected by them until they responded to specific questions about their sexual interests.[16]

The lack of visibility of the majority of the homosexually oriented is a major factor in a number of the problems associated with homosexuality:

First, it leads to a considerable underestimation of the size of the population who are to some degree homosexually oriented and thus reduces the impetus to deal with the range of problems encountered by this large population.

Second, society tends to generalize from the minority of homosexually oriented who *are* visible and thus stereotypes the entire population. Thus, the popular misconceptions are that homosexually oriented men are "effeminate," and the women are "masculine" and that most gays spend their time prowling after children or cruising in bars, baths, public bathrooms, and park bushes.

Third, those who are visible to the helping professions are generally those seeking help. Therefore, generalizations of many clinicians about homosexuality are based on a clinical sample which is not typical of the larger well-functioning populations.

Fourth, few if any, visible models are available to those homosexually oriented who are trying to develop coping strategies as individuals or as gay or lesbian couples.

Fifth, those growing up experiencing a homosexual preference feel isolated, alone and unique and have little opportunity in developing "pre-intimacy" experiences with others which would prepare them for more satisfying adult relationships.

Sixth, since invisibility provides some protection from societal sanctions against homosexuality, and there is little support for public labeling, homosexually oriented individuals must make many difficult decisions related to whether or not to make themselves visible ("coming out") and if so, to whom and how?

A major function of social work education, therefore, is to make homosexuality more visible. By so doing, stereotyping and fear of the unknown are reduced, leading the way to more effective interventions. The first step is an intensive exploration of the student's (and society's) need to label.

THE NEED TO LABEL

The use of the terms "homosexual" and "gay" can have profound effect upon those who label themselves or others. As noted in the discussion of reification and bifurcation, homosexuality is "commonly seen as a condition characterizing certain persons. . . . If homosexuality is a condition, then people either have it or do not have it."[17] Following this line of reasoning, a person *is* a homosexual or *is not* a homosexual. This labeling pressure reflects complex social influences which lead individuals to perceive themselves, and others as *either* "gay" or "straight." Our society (unlike others) has provided roles and prescribed behaviors for "gays" and "straights" but offers little reinforcement for those who don't accept or live according to *either* label. Those who don't accept either role are in a no man's (or woman's) land, reinforced by neither those who label themselves as "straight" nor those who label themselves as "gay." Consider, for example, the power of the epithet "closet queen" used against those who may have some degree of homosexual wishes or activity and have not accepted that social role or label.

Whether one perceives oneself as "straight" or "gay" is a result of complex learning procedures. Since homosexual behavior has been oppressed, a deviant role: gay, has emerged, along with certain prescribed role behaviors, which facilitate the daily functioning of some of those living within the role. Being gay, then, describes not only a sexual orientation but can lead to the assumption of an identity with a social group, complete with its own meeting places, argot, non-sexual as well as sexual role behaviors and even churches. These attributes which help clarify who is gay and who is not, are solidified by the rejection experienced by those who live within the gay subcultures from many of those within the prevalent straight community. While labeling simplifies the complexities of sexuality, it also obscures the wholeness of human beings.

PERCEPTIONS OF SEPARATENESS

In a class I taught at Berkeley, a leader of a local lesbian activist group spoke of her preference to have only lesbian friends, attend only lesbian bars, and, if possible, shop only in stores and eat only in restaurants owned and operated by lesbians. She said she encouraged her group members to do the same. She would just as soon have as little contact with straights as possible. The students in the class challenged this position, and felt it detrimental to mutual understanding and acceptance of members of gay and straight sub-cultures. A young black male student defended the woman's position and said he understood how she felt. As far as he was concerned, he chose to interact as little as possible with whites and had no desire to help whites understand or interact with blacks. The empathy of the black man for the gay woman led to a discussion of how some members of oppressed minorities respond to those who belong to the oppressing majority. There is often an understandable resentment, avoidance and depreciation of the majority group and the desire to stay with those with whom one identifies in important ways.

Members of some gay subcultures may agree with those in other oppressed minorities who suggest that professionals and researchers could more profitably turn their efforts at understanding themselves as members of the majority oppressing groups before they attempt to "understand" the behaviors of the oppressed minorities. The interest of majority group members is thus often suspect and those who offer to try to help may be rejected as "do-gooders," "professional liberals" and "voyeurs."

CONFUSION OVER THE SICKNESS LABEL

Whether or not to superimpose the sickness label on top of the homosexual label creates confusion for some students and practitioners. Many of those who have had no homosexual experiences or fantasies, as well as some who have, have learned to perceive homosexual behavior as evidence of mental illness.

Attitudes toward the constructs of "illness" applied to human behavior have changed radically in recent years. As behaviors are re-defined as either dysfunctional or functional rather than diseased or healthy, normal or abnormal, perceptions of sexual behavior have gone through a similar metamorphosis. As noted earlier, this change has been formalized by the revisions in the American Psychiatric Association's definition of homosexuality. That organization, in December 1973, removed "homosexuality" per se from the *Diagnostic and Statistical Manual of Psychiatric Disorders.*[18] In its place they substituted a new category "Sexual Orientation Disturbance" to describe "individuals whose sexual interests are directed primarily toward people of the same sex and who are either bothered by, in confict with, or wish to change their sexual orientation. This diagnostic category is distinguished from homosexuality which by itself does not constitute a psychiatric disorder."[19] (It must be observed that members of the gay subcultures may well view the APA action removing homosexuality as a disease with the same "relief" that Jews experienced from the papal decree of the same year absolving them of the responsibility for killing Jesus.)

By implication, then, a homosexual orientation is now officially considered a problem only if so defined by the individual experiencing it. It is significant and a bit frightening that this political decision by the APA can have a profound effect on the perceptions of—and ultimately the reactions to—the behavior and self-fulfillment of a sizable portion of our society. When all was said and done, the perceptions of the "illness" of homosexuality reduced itself to a social value and a political decision: one day an illness, the next day not.

Both the APA and the 1973 Delegate assembly of NASW have also passed resolutions deploring the deprivation of civil rights—and other forms of discrimination to those with homosexual orientations. The APA resolution "supports and urges the repeal of all legislation making criminal offenses of sexual acts performed by consenting adults in private."[20]

It is noteworthy that several religious bodies have either explored or passed resolutions decreasing religious sanctions against homosexual behavior. Such positions of official church bodies take time to filter down to and affect the attitudes of all church members. Despite these formal actions, the perception of homosexual behavior as either an "illness" and/or a "sin" persists in the minds of not only "mental health" practitioners, "straight" citizens and students, but many homosexually oriented people as well.

LEARNING EXPERIENCES

Based on the above observations of the problems social work students may have in understanding homosexuality, in practicing social work in relation to problems associated with homosexuality, and in combating oppressive elements in their community, a number of learning experiences have been helpful in social work classes and continuing education workshops taught by the author.

1. *Conceptualization of community attitudes which have created sexual oppression.* Students are presented with the concepts of the reproductive bias as a major factor (at least until the recent past) in influencing not only community sexual sanctions, but their own thinking about sexual behavior as well. In simple form, the reproductive bias suggests that the only good, moral, healthy, appropriate, productive, natural, normal (etc.) sexual activities are those which could conceivably (pun intended) lead to socially approved pregnancies. Although this bias works against the sexual fulfillment of a number of groups to a greater or lesser extent, the homosexually oriented are among the most victimized. Homosexual behavior cannot conceivably lead to *any* pregnancy, let alone a socially approved one, and it therefore violates the popular conception of acceptable sexuality.

While the reproductive bias may have been functional when any population's strength was measured by its ratio of births to population, the bias has become increasingly non-functional as over-population has become a more common concern. The greater acceptance of homosexuality in our culture may indeed reflect a growing acceptance of the desirability of separating sexuality from reproduction.

Other factors have certainly contributed in the past to the bias against homosexual behavior including for example, the application of the work ethic to sexuality: sex is acceptable as long as it's functional[21] but the reproductive bias is probably among the most significant influences.

2. *Direct contact with members of "gay" sub-cultures.* Many graduate students have never knowingly met individuals who are primarily homosexually oriented or who are members of gay sub-cultures. It is useful to expose social work students to a wide range of homosexually oriented individuals in order to humanize the concept. Educational research has shown that exposure to homosexu-

ally oriented men and women in classroom units on homosexuality is effective in reducing negative stereotyping.[22,23]

Whenever possible, both men and women of various ages, ethnic groups, and those living in diverse life styles are included. In classes given by the author, gay couples, ministers, social workers, currently and formerly married individuals, mothers, fathers, and individuals who enjoy sex with both men and women, have spoken to large classes as well as serving as resource persons in small groups.

Often these presentations are part of a panel organized to follow a series of films portraying explicit sexual behavior. In this way, the students are able to integrate or at least confront their feelings about specific homosexual activities and the particular human beings they are "meeting" and perhaps empathizing with in class. Generally, the panel responds first to prepared questions from me which anticipate some of the students' more frequent areas of concern. Some of these questions are: "If you could take a free 'magic pill' which would convert you to a heterosexual orientation and it had no side effects, would you take it?" (Generally, no. But they might if it had been offered to them as adolescents.) "Do you know what caused you to be homosexually oriented?" (No, do you know what caused you to be heterosexual?) "What do you do in bed?" (It depends on what I and my partner feel like doing.) Throughout this discussion, an attempt is made to avoid heaviness, to encourage humor and to bring out the uniqueness and humanness of each of the panel. Then, students are invited to ask their own questions, and, after class, to join the panel at the campus beer hall.

In addition to panels, gay organizations have sponsored parties in members' homes for social work students, and acted as their hosts to local bars. Many students report that such experiences radically change their stereotypes, reduce their own anxieties, and at the same time begin to make them aware of the diverse characteristics of life within the various gay sub-cultures. Some students have also reported that these experiences make them more comfortable and less defensive about their own sexual orientations.

3. *Formal research.* A number of students have met the MSW research requirements through studies of the characteristics and problems experienced by diverse gay sub-cultures. One study[24] explored the relationships of male gay couples who have lived to-

gether for at least a year. This sample of 20 couples was found to be essentially very well functioning. The couples tended to be well-educated, in their thirties, with good incomes. Their relationships were not divided into traditional male-female roles. Sexual satisfaction and activities were perceived as a relatively minor factor relationships: love was a major factor. They noted that both the gay and straight communities discouraged permanent relationships, and shared some anxieties about ultimate effects of the pressures on their relationships.

It was noteworthy that while some couples reported difficulties in their relationships or anticipated the possibilities of such difficulties, they would not see any of the "mental health" professions or agencies as a resource for help. If they did seek help, they felt another gay person would be in the best position to understand and help them.

Presentations of such research findings to classes emphasize both the diversity of such life styles often loosely subsumed under "homosexuality" in addition to the scope of services social workers could provide.[25]

4. *Viewing explicit sexual films.* Students report that the viewing of explicit, well-produced films of homosexual relationships and homosexual activity facilitates exploring and coping with their own emotional reactions.[26] While part of the purpose of showing these films is to desensitize students to homosexual behavior, and to inform them of a range of homosexual activities, they have the broader purpose of exposing students to their own feeling about homosexual behavior.

"After the Game" is an example of a film which has been useful in exploring a variety of issues. Two young, attractive women who perceive themselves as heterosexually oriented find themselves in a situation in which they must deal with their erotic feelings for each other and the consequent anxiety about self-labelling. This film initiates considerable discussion about the continuum of sexual orientation and the power of labels. As with many of the films shown, however, students also explore some of the filmmakers' biases. For example, this film reinforces the stereotype that women turn to each other sexually and emotionally only because of bad experiences with insensitive men.

Reactions to these films, of course, are as diverse as the students who watch them. Typical responses range from "I could take all that genital stuff, but the affection between these people—like the handholding and the kissing—repulsed me" to "I got turned on by watching what they did, and I think that's all right, even though I wouldn't necessarily want to do it myself."

5. *Watching and discussing current movies and popular commercial television.* Students are urged to see and discuss current movies and television programs which include homosexually oriented characters. Within the last few years there have been a number of such presentations which include individuals whose sexual orientation and life patterns are more complex than former stereotypes.

Many of these dramatizations reflect an awareness of life styles and concerns experienced by people who do not necessarily identify with a gay subculture. Recently students have seen and evaluated their reactions to "Personal Best," "Making Love," "Deathtrap," and such plays as "Find Your Way Home," "5th of July," "Chorus Line" and "Torch Song Trilogy." Classic films such as "The Sergeant," "Sunday Bloody Sunday," "The Fox," and the television film "That Certain Summer" are also remembered by some and discussed. While some of these fictional presentations disturb some students, they all can be seen as valuable mirrors of the values of at least a segment of the population at the time in which they are made. Movies such as "Cruising," "Taxi to the Toilet," and "Making Love" also provide an opportunity to discuss reactions to particular gay subcultures.

The popular television evening soap opera series "Dynasty" led to an exploration of society's current ambivalence toward homosexuality. When the series was first introduced in 1980, a major character was homosexually oriented. He was portrayed as an attractive, intelligent, sensitive and thoroughly miserable human being. He had had a lover who didn't really turn him on, and subsequently left him. He then went to bed with a friend's wife, realized that he was basically heterosexually oriented, fell passionately in love with a young woman, married her. She subsequently left him, and in the next television season, the character was removed.

6. *Provision of information regarding medical, legal and religious aspects of homosexuality.* Content on homosexuality should include current information about the medical, legal and religious aspects of sexuality.

Homosexual activities require an understanding of the physical expression of sexual desire. The range of homosexual expression can be explored with the understanding that the specific nature of sexual expression chosen varies among individuals and over time. Also, an understanding of the nature, symptoms and treatment of sexually transmitted diseases should be explored, including emerging knowledge about acquired immunodeficiency syndrome (AIDS), which contributes to such potentially fatal diseases as Kaposi's sarcoma and pneumocystis carinii pneumonia. Epidemiologists from the STD programs can be invited to discuss the current knowledge regarding such diseases. The psychological impact of AIDS as a life-threatening consequence of sexual activity cannot be minimized. It has already had to impact on the sexual behavior of many homosexually oriented individuals.

Legal issues related to homosexuality should also be explored. Approximately half the states in the U.S.A. still have laws against homosexual acts even between consenting adults in private. There is a complex web of local laws related to homosexual activities and the rights of homosexually oriented individuals in such areas as employment and housing. There are also a number of legal concerns regarding the right of partners in gay and lesbian couples as well as problems in relation to custody of children of gay and lesbian individuals. Law professors, family court staff, and police representatives can be called upon to review and explain local and state legislation and enforcement related to homosexuality.

Finally, many social work clients and students are concerned with interpretations of religious stands on homosexuality. There is much confusion over just what the Bible has to say about homosexuality (for example, just what did Jesus say about homosexuality? answer: nothing). While there seems to be almost endless debates about biblical statements concerning homosexuality, some recent biblical scholars[27] have put such debates into clearer perspective. In addition to reviewing the recent publications of biblical scholars and statements from various national religious denominations, it might be useful to invite a range of religious practitioners to explore religious opinions related to homosexuality and then discuss the relation, and potential conflicts, of various religious beliefs about homosexuality with social work values.

7. *Presentations of specific interventive needs and procedures*. Knowledge related to homosexual behavior and gay subcultures, along with the exploration of feelings and attitudes about homosexual behavior are requisites to a worthwhile discussion of interventive goals and procedures. For example, as a result of this foundation, discussion of treatment facilitating heterosexual activi-

ties becomes only one approach as a possible alternative available to those clients who want it. Considerably more time is used on consideration of community education, social system change, resource development and special counseling needs to facilitate free sexual choice.

Students are introduced to a variety of potential problems and treatment considerations. Social workers, for example, can be effective in helping individuals who are coming out to consider the various options for gay life styles, and to make decisions about what, if anything to tell whom (e.g., parents, gay and straight friends, employers, etc.) how and when. If the individual is heterosexually married, both partners may be involved in a decision-making process about the marriage, and the nature of their future relationship with each other and any children. The special problems of the spouses, children and parents of the homosexually oriented should be explored.[28]

Partners in ongoing gay relationships may seek help in a role relationship which, for many, is difficult to maintain in response to a constellation of social forces. Helping couples develop clear communication in their relationships, and strategies to cope with jealousy related to outside relationships can help overcome problems commonly encountered in gay couples. Students can also explore recent findings about the stages of gay couple relationships and the range of problems commonly encountered at each stage.[29]

Many homosexually oriented, divorced, or unmarried women experience considerable pressures in keeping and raising children. Social workers can help as their advocate in surmounting legal and bureaucratic obstacles to their parenting. There are also specific problems encountered by adolescents who experience homosexual feelings and consider themselves unique and "freakish." At the other end of the age spectrum are aging men and women who may feel "nobody loves you when you are old and gay!"[30]

On a broader scale, social workers individually and collectively can facilitate in "delabelling" homosexuality as in illness and crime, and thus help to decrease the unnecessary suffering associated with homosexual choice and behavior. There are states which still have legislation against homosexual behavior, cities in which homosexuals are harassed or worse, entrapped into homosexual offenses, and locations in which gay couples cannot rent apartments. In areas in which such problems occur, class time (and perhaps field experiences) can be used to consider the application of various social work roles to such problems. Policies of social agencies may also be explored as they relate to the needs and rights of gay and lesbian clients and staff, "people in glass houses."

The emphasis in teaching an approach to those who are homosexually oriented should take into consideration the trend in social work in which the focus of intervention is shifting from treating those who are different to conform, to supporting their rights, including their rights to be different.[31] I believe that this is the intent of the new curriculum policy statement of the Council on Social Work Education, effective July 1, 1983:

> Special Populations: The social work profession, by virtue of its system of ethics, its traditional value commitments, and its long history of work in the whole range of human services, is committed to preparing students to understand and appreciate cultural and social diversity. The profession has also been concerned about the consequences of oppression...The curriculum...should include content on other special population groups...in particular, groups that have been consistently affected by social, economic and legal bias or oppression. Such groups include those distinguished by age, religions, disablement, sexual orientation and culture."[32]

This paper has attempted to present some ideas on how that content may be conceptualized and presented in social work education.

REFERENCES

1. Gochros, H. "Teaching More or Less Straight Social Work Students to be Helpful to More or Less Gay People," *The Homosexual Counseling Journal*, Vol. 2 No. 2 April 1975.

2. See Gochros, H. "Introducing Human Sexuality into the Graduate Social Work Curriculum," *Social Work Education Reporter*, September 1970; "Human Sexuality in the Social Work Curriculum" SIECUS REPORT (Sex Information & Education Council of the U.S.), November 1972, p. 6; Gene Johnson, "A Study of Sex Education in the Schools of Social Work," University of Washington, 1972, and Leigh Hallingby, "Human Sexuality in the Social Work Education Curriculum at the University of Pennsylvania," University of Pennsylvania, 1972, unpublished MSW research projects.

3. McWhirter, D. and Matteson, D., *The Male Couple*. Englewood Cliffs: New Jersey, Prentice Hall; 1983.

4. Gochros, H. *op. cit.*

5. Gochros, H. "The Sexually Oppressed," *Social Work,* March 1972, Vol. 17, No. 2, pp. 16-23.

6. Tully, Carol, and Albro, Joyce C., "Homosexuality: A Social Worker's Imbroglio," *Journal of Sociology and Social Welfare,* March 1979, Vol. 6, No. 2.

(see also) Gochros, H. and Ricketts, W. "Homosexual Clients," in Yelaja, S. *Ethical Issues in Social Work.* Springfield Illinois: Charles C. Thomas, 1982.

7. Levitt, E. and Klasser, A. "Public Attitudes Toward Homosexuality," *Journal of Homosexuality,* 1974, Vol. 1, pp. 30-32.

8. Davison, G. and Wilson, G. T. "Attitudes of Behavior Therapists Toward Homosexuality," *Behavior Therapy,* 4:690, 1973.

9. Masters, W.H. and Johnson, V.E. *Homosexuality in Perspective.* Boston: Little, Brown Co. 1979.

10. Garfinkle, E.M. and Morin, S.F. "Psychologists' Attitudes Toward Homosexual Psychotherapy Clients," *Journal of Social Issues,* 34(3):109, 1978.

11. Brown, D. "Counseling the Youthful Homosexual," *The School Counselor,* p. 330, 1975.

12. Zilbergeld, B. *Male Sexuality: A Guide to Sexual Fulfillment.* Boston, Little, Brown Co., 1978.

13. Focault, M. *The History of Sexuality.* New York; Pantheon Books, 1978, p. 43.

14. Kinsey, A., Pomeroy, W.B., and Martin, C.E. *Sexual Behavior in the Human Male.* Philadelphia: W.B. Saunders, Co., 1948.
For a comparison with a contemporary survey of the incidence of homosexuality in a representative large sample, see also:
Hunt, M. "Sexual Behavior in the 1970's, Part VI: Deviant Sexuality," *Playboy,* March 1974, pp. 54-55.

15. Thomas, W.I. *Social Behavior and Personality.* New York: Social Science Research Council, 1951, p. 81.

16. Pomeroy, W. *Personal Communication at the Institute for Advanced Studies of Human Sexuality,* San Francisco, 1979.

17. McIntosh, M. "The Homosexual Role," *Social Problems,* 1968, Vol. 16, p. 183.

18. "Proceedings of the Board of Trustees of the American Psychiatric Association" December 1973.

19. *Ibid.*

20. *Ibid.*

21. See for example, Lewis, L. and Brissett, D., "Sex as Work: A Study of Advocational Counseling," *Social Problems,* Summer 1967, Vol. 15, No.1, pp. 8-18 and Johnson, V. and Masters, W. "Contemporary Influences on Sexual Response: The Work Ethic." Paper presented at the Second Annual SIECUS Citation Dinner, October 18, 1972, New York.

22. Greenberg, J.S. "A Study of Personality Change Associated with the Conducting of a High School Unit on Homosexuality," *The Journal of School of Health,* VLV (7):394-398, September 1975.

23. Morin, S.F. "Educational Programs as a Means of Changing Attitudes Toward Gay People," *Homosexual Counseling Journal,* 1(4):160-165, October 1974.

24. Columbia, J., DeWolfe, V., Fitch, V., and Reimer, L., *Gay Male Couples in Hawaii.* Unpublished Master's Project, University of Hawaii School of Social Work, May 1973.

25. One student who came out while in graduate school went on to help establish a community oriented counseling and education service for sexual minorities in a large urban area. Another student introduced free VD screening and counseling at the local gay baths.

26. Films found to be especially effective are "Holding" (female couple) and "Vir Amat" (male couple) produced and distributed by Multi Media, San Francisco; and Gene Genet's "Le Chant d'Amour" (male homosexual relationship in a French prison) available through Evergreen Films, New York and "Gender" (transvestite/song) and "After the

Game" (ambiguous relationship between two women) available through Focus International Films, New York City.

27. Boswell, J., *Christianity, Social Tolerance and Homosexuality*. Chicago; University of Chicago Press, 1980.

28. See for example:

> Miller, M., "Homosexual Husbands: What Wives Must Know," *Redbook*, April 1975.
>
> Kohn, B., Matusow, A., *Barry and Alice: Portrait of a Bisexual Marriage*. Prentice Hall, 1980.
>
> Hobson, L.Z., *Consenting Adult*. Warner Paperback, 1976.

29. McWhirter and Matteson. *op. cit.*

30. Berger, R.M. *Gay and Gray*. Urbana, Illinois; University of Illinois Press, 1982.

31. Kittrie, N., *The Right to be Different: Deviance and Enforced Therapy*. Baltimore: Johns Hopkins, 1972.

> see also:

Dulaney, D.D., and Kelly, J., "Improving Services to Gay and Lesbian Clients," *Social Work*, Vol. 27, No. 2, March 1982.

32. Council on Social Work Education, *Curriculum Policy for The Masters Degree and Baccalaureate Degree Programs in Social Work Education*. New York. C.S.W.E., 1982.